Home Health Care Answer Book

Legal Issues for Providers

Martha Dale Nathanson, EdS, JD
*Director
Risk Management and
Regulatory Affairs
for Home Health
Kirson Medical
Baltimore, Maryland*

An Aspen Publication®
Aspen Publishers, Inc.
Gaithersburg, Maryland
1995

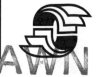

This publication is designed to provide accurate and authoritative information in regard to the Subject Matter covered. It is sold with the understanding that the publisher is not engaged in rendering legal, accounting, or other professional service. If legal advice or other expert assistance is required, the service of a competent professional person should be sought. *(From a Declaration of Principles jointly adopted by a Committee of the American Bar Association and a Committee of Publishers and Associations.)*

Library of Congress Cataloging-in-Publication Data
Nathanson, Martha Dale
Home health care answer book : legal issues for providers / Martha Dale Nathanson.
p.   cm.
Includes bibliographical references and index.
ISBN: 0-8342-0575-0
1. Home care services—Law and legislation—United States. I. Title.
KF3826.H64N38   1995
344.73′03214—dc20
[347.3043214]
94-43448
CIP

Editorial Resources: Ruth Bloom

Library of Congress Catalog Card Number: 94-43448
ISBN: 0-8342-0575-0

Printed in the United States of America

1   2   3   4   5

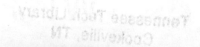

Table of Contents _____

Introduction

The Home Health Care Answer Book is designed for administrators, clinical personnel, employment managers, and investors who need direct answers and general information about the legal questions they encounter in the day-to-day operation of their home health agencies. Given the rapid growth of the home care industry and its integration into larger health care delivery systems, *The Home Health Care Answer Book* will also be useful for other types of health care providers such as physicians and hospitals, as well as payers such as insurers and health maintenance organizations, all of whom provide for the home care needs of their patients. Professionals such as attorneys, accountants, and business advisors will also benefit from using this resource as they address questions from their home care clients.

The Home Health Care Answer Book addresses the home health agency as a specialized health care provider, an employer, a billing entity, and as a business engaging in the normal range of contractual and operational activities. It addresses laws and regulations at both the federal and state levels. As a general guide to the array of legal issues affecting the home health agency, it serves as a quick reference to give the reader a working knowledge of those issues, and directs the reader to sources that provide even more detail about their problem. The user may find it useful to peruse *The Home Health Care Answer Book* as a whole, to become familiar with the types of problems they may encounter, or to review possible solutions to the many problems they may have already encountered.

The book's ultimate appeal is in the ease with which the reader can find answers to specific questions that are certain to arise.

The Home Health Care Answer Book could not have been written without the contributions of several individuals. Diane Pederson, Executive Director of the Maryland Association for Home Care, reviewed the manuscript for clinically related content, and Annette N. DeBois, an attorney in private practice in Albuquerque, New Mexico, reviewed it for business-related issues. Special thanks go to Donald M. Kirson, Robert J. O'Connor, and Robert Murphy of Kirson Medical Equipment Co., and to James D'Orta, MD, Medical Advisor to Kirson Medical Equipment Co., for their insight into the changes affecting the home care market and the operational challenges arising as a result of these changes.

Martha D. Nathanson, Esq.

List of Questions _____

1—Overview of Home Health Care

2—Licenses and Other Permits To Operate

Overview of Regulatory Permits

Licensure of Home Health Agencies

Certificate of Need for Home Health Agencies

3—Business-Related Legal Issues

Forms of Legal Organization

Bankruptcy Law

Antitrust Law

4—Contracting for Services

Contracting for Ancillary Services

Managed Care Contracting

5—Employment Issues

Hiring Staff

Employment at Will

Negligent Hiring

Independent Contractors Versus Employees

Employment Contracts

Covenants Not To Compete

Employment Discrimination

Title VII of the Civil Rights Act

Drug Testing of Employees

The Family and Medical Leave Act

Employee Compensation

Safety

6—Medicare Reimbursement

Conditions of Participation

Conditions of Coverage

7—Patient Care Issues

Abuse and Neglect

Consent

Advance Directives

Surrogate Decisionmaking

"Do Not Resuscitate" Orders

Guardianship of Disabled or Incompetent Persons

Patient Abandonment

8—Recordkeeping

1

Overview of Home Health Care

Q.1:1 What is home health care?

Home health care refers to the provision of medical and related services in a noninstitutional or residential setting. This setting is usually the patient's home but may just as easily be the home of a relative or family friend. It may also be a nursing home if that is the patient's residence and the nursing home does not provide the necessary skilled care.

The types of care that may be provided in the home include

- skilled nursing;
- custodial care;
- home medical equipment services;
- respiratory and ventilator services, including oxygen therapy;
- infusion therapy;
- physical, occupational, or speech therapy;
- home health aide services; and
- medical social work services.

Q.1:2 What are some of the essential characteristics of home health care that differentiate it from care given in an institutional environment?

The primary difference between health care delivered in the home and care delivered in an institutional setting such as a hospital or

1

skilled nursing facility is the lack of the continuous presence of professional health care providers. Hospitals are staffed with physicians and nurses who monitor the patient on-site, and various types of equipment are available at all times to indicate when emergency situations must be addressed.

In the home care setting, however, the primary monitors of care are the family members or friends who attend the patient. The care is monitored by professionals off-site as often as it is through visits to the patient. The main difference is the patient's need for a professional to be on-site and the frequency of such monitoring. In home care, frequent monitoring of the patient by the family or caregiver is communicated to the home care professional by telephone, and the professional can then make a clinical decision as to whether a visit is appropriate.

In addition, home care is not provided in a single site. The medical professionals are all in different locations, and the patient is in yet a third location. Therefore, the need for structured communication procedures is even more critical than in the institutional setting.

Q.1:3 What are the characteristics of the typical users of home health care services?

Home health care is appropriate for a broad range of people in very different situations. Approximately 2.5 percent of the American population received home health care from an agency of some sort, according to a 1987 survey. About half of the recipients were over age 65. [See *Basic Statistics about Home Care*, National Association for Home Care, p. 5, reprinting National Medical Expenditures Survey, 1987.] The top five diagnoses of home care patients upon discharge from the hospital are stroke, chronic obstructive pulmonary disease, heart failure, major joint procedures, and hip/femur procedures. [See *Basic Statistics about Home Care*, National Association for Home Care, p. 6, reprinting "Medicare Patients and Postacute Care: Who Goes Where?" Rand Corporation, 1989.] Nearly one-quarter of the patients receiving home care suffer from circulatory disorders. [See *Basic Statistics about Home Care*, National Association for Home Care, p. 6, reprinting NCHS Sample Survey, 1992.] In addition, individuals of any age recovering from surgery or managing a chronic disease, such as cancer or AIDS, may use home health services.

Pediatric patients constitute a growing population of consumers of home health services, including newborns, who may receive home phototherapy services for bilirubin; young cancer patients receiving chemotherapy; and children receiving intravenous antibiotic treatment for intractable infections. Any of these individuals might in the past have received some portion of needed care in an inpatient setting. As the locus of care moves from the hospital to alternate sites, the market for home care services will continue to grow.

Q.1:4 What is a home health service?

Home health service is a term found in many state statutes that define the particular kinds of services that may or may not be provided by a home health agency. For example, home health services in Illinois are defined as "services provided to a person at his residence according to a plan of treatment for illness or infirmity prescribed by a physician. Such services include part time and intermittent nursing services, and other therapeutic services such as physical therapy, occupational therapy, speech therapy, medical social services, or services provided by a home health aide."

Q.1:5 What is a home health agency?

Home health agency is a term with specific meaning; not all of the services provided in the home are viewed as provided by a home health agency (HHA). Generally, a home health agency is defined as a "private or public organization, including, but not limited to, any partnership, corporation, political subdivision of the state, or other government agency within the state, which provides, or arranges for the provision of, skilled nursing services, to persons in their temporary or permanent place of residence." [Cal. Health and Safety Code §1727(a).]

Other states include much more as provided by an HHA. In Texas, an HHA is a place of business, including a hospice, that provides a home health service. [See preceding question.] In Illinois, an HHA is defined as "a public agency or private organization that provides skilled nursing services and at least one other home health service." [See preceding question.]

In an interesting development reflecting a tighter scope of regulation, Texas, in 1993, broadened the definition of *home health agency*. It replaced the term *health* with the term *and community support services*. These extra services include "hospice or personal assistance services for pay or other consideration in a client's residence, an independent living environment, or another appropriate location."

Q.1:6 What services are generally provided by an HHA?

The central service provided by an HHA is skilled nursing, that is, "services provided by a registered nurse or licensed vocational nurse." [Cal. Health and Safety Code §1727(b).] The HHA usually provides home health aide services as well. These home health aide services must be provided by "a person certified by the state department to provide these services." [Cal. Health and Safety Code §1727(c).] However, some states only recently included home health aides or attendant care. [See Texas Health and Safety Chapter 142.001(5).]

Q.1:7 What about other services provided in the home?

Other types of services provided in the home may or may not be provided by HHAs, depending upon the state law or upon business practice. For example, most HHAs do not provide home medical equipment (HME), but rather contract with an HME company to provide those services to their patients. In some states, infusion therapy; oxygen therapy; nurse registry services; hospice services; physical, occupational, and speech therapy; and social work services are provided by home health agencies, while in other states they are not. [See Texas Stat. Ann. Health and Safety Chapter 142, which includes all of these services in its definition of an HHA.] The rule of thumb is if a service is not expressly identified as such, it is not considered a home health service.

Q.1:8 What is a Medicare-certified HHA?

A certified HHA is one that is certified by an official of the Department of Health and Human Services as in compliance with the conditions of participation in Title XVIII Social Security Act. [42 U.S.C. §§1395 *et seq.*] Medicare-certified HHAs are the only HHAs that can receive reimbursement for home health services provided to Medicare beneficiaries.

Q.1:9 What are the two major types of HHAs?

The two major types of HHAs are hospital or institutional based and free-standing. Traditionally, a hospital-based HHA was usually a department of the hospital. More recently, however, it is common for a hospital and HHA to enter into a joint venture to develop an HHA or bring the HHA into an overall integrated delivery system of which the hospital is the central element.

Q.1:10 What types of legal issues are likely to arise in the running of a home health business?

Several types of legal issues affect home health providers. As with any business, contractual obligations for providing and receiving services must be met. Criminal sanctions may apply for violation of statutory provisions covering delivery of services and reimbursement or for failure to report abuse or neglect. Additionally, regulatory requirements not necessarily involving criminal sanctions present numerous legal issues relating to, for example, certificate of need, reimbursement, and licensure. An HHA owes each patient a duty of reasonable care, and this could be violated through a failure to keep medical records confidential, through a failure to get proper consent, and through negligence in the delivery of health care services. Business-related issues, such as employment, taxation, bankruptcy, and antitrust issues, also affect the operation of a home health agency.

Q.1:11 How are HHAs regulated?

HHAs are regulated under federal, state, and local law. For example, federal laws such as Medicare, the Bankruptcy Act, the Fair Labor Standards Act, Title VII of the Civil Rights Act of 1964, and the Occupational Safety and Health Act apply to home health agencies. At the state level, an HHA would have to consider the licensure of the agency, the possible need for the agency to obtain a CON, and the licensure status of its professional employees.

Local laws such as taxation, zoning, and business registration laws must also be considered. Finally, the HHA's standards of quality may be measured against standards developed by an accrediting organization such as the Joint Commission on Accreditation of Healthcare Organizations (Joint Commission). Although accreditation is voluntary, accreditation standards influence the oversight of the home health industry by other regulatory entities.

Q.1:12 What national and state associations address the needs of HHAs?

The four major national associations that address home care nursing issues are the National Association for Home Care, Visiting Nurse Association of America, Home Health Services and Staffing Association, and American Federation of Home Health Agencies. In addition, most states have a state-based home care association, which may or may not be an affiliate of one of the national groups. Many states also have state groups representing providers of hospice services, home IV therapy services, and durable medical equipment services.

In some states, the home health association and other associations addressing home care issues are beginning to coordinate efforts and share resources. For example, Tennessee's home health association and the home medical equipment association have recently merged, and associations in other states are following this lead. The associations find that by combining their resources they can address industry developments such as legislative initiatives, reimbursement changes, and personnel issues more efficiently and effectively.

2

Licenses and Other Permits To Operate

Home health services, like other health care services, must meet certain standards in order to ensure that the care delivered is of a certain quality. State health departments are mandated to safeguard the health and safety of state residents and have developed regulatory systems that articulate the standards of quality that health care providers must meet. The primary method by which a home health agency is determined to be qualified to deliver care in the state is through the licensure process. In reviewing an agency's application for a license to operate, the state will examine the agency's resources and policies and grant the license if appropriate.

In addition, home health care is but one aspect of a state's or a region's health care resources. A home health agency's services must complement the health care services in the area. In deciding whether or not a particular service is needed, a state must balance its available resources against its needs and allocate those resources carefully. This allocation is embodied in the certificate-of-need process, a process that is undergoing great change. Yet even in jurisdictions where a CON may no longer be required, the concept remains a basic operational issue for the home health agency, as the standards developed through the years of the CON process have found their way into other regulatory schemes developed by states to manage their health care resources.

OVERVIEW OF REGULATORY PERMITS

Q.2:1 What types of authority may an HHA need to operate in a particular jurisdiction?

An HHA may need either a license, a certificate, or a registration to operate in any given area. In addition, accreditation by an association may be required, or at least desirable, in some instances. The differences between the three types of credentials are often blurred, as states vary in the terms they use to describe the process of overseeing the establishment of health care entities. A brief discussion of each type is, however, appropriate.

Licensure generally applies to professional activities and the performance of such activities. A license is defined as the "authority or permission to do or carry on some trade or business which would otherwise be unlawful." [*Black's Law Dictionary*, 5th ed., West Publishing Co., 1979.] Thus, health care professionals with professional types of duties are required to obtain licenses to practice. For example, physicians, nurses, therapists, attorneys, and health care administrators would need to obtain licenses. Usually the licensure process involves thorough courses of study in preparation for taking comprehensive examinations that test not only the applicants' memory of rules and concepts but their ability to apply those in particular situations using their professional skills.

Certification is defined as "a written assurance, or official representation that some act has or has not been done, some legal formality complied with." [*Black's Law Dictionary*, 5th ed., West Publishing Co., 1979.] While similar to licensure, it more closely represents an acknowledgment of the individual's or entity's accomplishment of certain tasks or goals rather than the application of specific professional knowledge. Thus, a nursing home surveyor would be certified by the state, or a benefits administrator would be certified by an association. The preparation may not be as comprehensive as that required for licensure.

Registration is the least involved of all of the forms of regulation by a state. *Black's Law Dictionary* defines registration as "the recording, enrolling, entering into an official register." [*Black's Law Dictionary*, 5th ed., West Publishing Co., 1979.] Thus, one can safely assume that a requirement to register as an HHA in a state, if such a requirement exists in any state, will not be difficult to comply with. In most instances, the process will involve simply filling in a form that asks for little more than ministerial information such as name, address, etc., and paying a registration fee. There will be no testing or survey, and thus the process does not provide substantive assurance that the entity provides quality services.

Finally, accreditation is a process through which a professional or trade association applies the standards developed for the delivery of services by its industry. This is a voluntary process, although in some industries the market demands only accredited providers. In addition, in some states, accreditation by an association will suffice for certification by the state, thus eliminating the need for two survey and certification processes. In the home health industry, the Joint Commission on Accreditation of Healthcare Organizations (Joint Commission) accredits home health agencies as well as equipment providers. In addition, the National League for Nursing's Community Health Accreditation Program (CHAP) accredits home health agencies.

LICENSURE OF HOME HEALTH AGENCIES

Q.2:2 What types of licenses are required to operate an HHA?

Some states require a specific license to operate an HHA. An HHA is also subject to local business licensure laws. In some states, a Medicare-certified HHA will obtain a different type of license than a noncertified agency. [See Texas Health and Safety Code Ann. §142 (West 1992).]

Q.2:3 What is the purpose of licensure for HHAs?

State statutes generally speak of licensure as the means by which the state can ensure the health and safety of the people of the state. Further, they mandate the state department of health to work to establish high standards of quality for home health agencies. [Cal.

Health and Safety Code §1725 (West 1990).] These standards are typically set through regulations developed by the state department of health. [See Md. Regs. Code Tit. X, §10.07.10 (1991).]

Q.2:4 What services are generally provided by an HHA?

Most HHAs provide skilled nursing care; occupational, physical, and speech therapy; and home health aide services. In addition, some HHAs provide custodial care or companionship services, home medical equipment services, infusion therapy, and oxygen therapy.

Q.2:5 What services are typically not provided by an HHA and can therefore be offered by an entity not licensed as an HHA?

In many states, entities that provide hospice services do not need HHA licensure. Also, nurse registries often do not need HHA licensure, as they do not provide any health care services themselves but function merely as employment or referral sources. [Cal. Health and Safety Code §1726 (West 1990).]

The typical types of services and the types of practitioners who provide them are described in the Texas statute as exempt from licensure:

- a physician, dentist, registered nurse, or physical therapist licensed under the Texas law, who provides home health services only as a part of and incidental to their private office practice;
- a registered nurse, licensed vocational nurse, physical therapist, occupational therapist, speech therapist, medical social worker, or any other health care professional who provides home health services as a sole practitioner;
- a nonprofit registry operated by a national or state professional association or society of licensed health care practitioners, that

operates solely as a clearinghouse to put consumers in contact with licensed health care practitioners who give care in a patient's residence and that does not maintain official patient records or direct patient services;

- an individual who resides permanently at the patient's residence;
- an employee of a person or entity licensed under this chapter;
- any home or institution for the disabled or elderly that provides health services only to its residents;
- a person who provides one health service through a contract with a person licensed under this chapter;
- a durable medical equipment supply company;
- a pharmacy or wholesale medical supply company that does not furnish services, other than supplies, to a person at the person's house;
- a hospital or other licensed health care facility that services only inpatient residents;
- a person providing home health services to an injured employee under the workers' compensation program; and
- a visiting nurse service conducted by and for adherents of a well-recognized church or religious denomination, and which furnishes nursing care only by prayer or spiritual means.

[Texas Health and Safety Code Ann. §142.003 (West 1992).]

Some states have attempted to fill in gaps left by such broad exemptions in their home health agency statutes. For example, Maryland's home health agency statute does not cover practice in the home setting by occupational therapists, speech therapists, physical therapists, audiologists, and other professionals who are licensed individually as professional practitioners. Thus, Maryland recently enacted a separate statute that covers the aspects of their practice that may qualify as home care but were unregulated as such. A practitioner who provides home treatment must register as a Residential Service Agency. [See Md. Code Ann. Health General Article §19-4A.]

Q.2:6 What regulatory body issues the necessary licenses?

All states have state departments of health that implement the requirements in the state's law relating to health care. These departments issue the licenses for HHAs. In addition, most states have a specific department that deals with the licensing of health care practitioners and facilities. This division oversees the application process and performs surveys to ensure that HHAs comply with all of the requirements in the pertinent laws and regulations.

Q.2:7 How long do HHA licenses last?

Typically, a license for a home health agency will last for one year. It may be renewed each year by mail, with verification of the name, address, and principals of the agency and submission of the required annual fee. Some jurisdictions may require an inspection after a number of years, and some of those jurisdictions may accept accreditation of the agency by a nationally recognized organization, typically the Joint Commission, as a substitute for state inspection. If accreditation is accepted as sufficient for automatic licensure, an accredited HHA is said to have "deemed status," i.e, the HHA is deemed to have met the requirements of the state by virtue of its having been accredited by the Joint Commission.

Q.2:8 What is the process for obtaining an HHA license?

The HHA submits an application to the department, arranges for an inspection, and pays the fee required in the statute. The application must provide the following information before it can be approved:

- documentation evidencing that the applicant has adequate financial resources to provide the services it is applying to provide during the term of the license;
- a list of all personnel and their qualifications and a plan for providing continuing training and education for those personnel during the term of the license;

- documentation establishing that the applicant can meet quality of care standards set by the department;
- the general service area and quantity and nature of the patient load;
- a plan for the orderly transfer of patients or provision of care to the patients by another provider if the HHA cannot, for any reason, maintain or deliver the services it has been authorized to deliver under the terms of the license;
- a plan for the establishment of a clinical recordkeeping system that meets the requirements set out by either the state or accreditation organizations;
- arrangements for the supervision of licensed and unlicensed personnel by a registered nurse or physical, speech, or occupational therapist when the services are performed within the therapist's scope of practice; and
- policies and procedures regarding the delivery and supervision of patient care and arrangements for regular review and revision, if necessary, of those policies by a group of professional personnel that includes a physician and registered nurse.

[See Texas Health and Safety Code Ann. §142.003 (West 1992); Cal. Health and Safety Code §1727.5; Illinois Ann. ch. 210 ¶55/2.05 *et seq.*]

Q.2:9 What are the fees for obtaining an HHA license?

The fees vary from state to state and are usually set annually by the legislature. For example, the fee for obtaining a license in Illinois is $25, and in Texas the fee is $526 for the main office and each branch. The fee for registration as a residential service agency in Maryland is $500.

Q.2:10 What types of inspections may the state department of health demand a home health agency undergo when the agency is applying for or already has a license?

The department of health, or its authorized representatives, may enter the premises of an HHA at reasonable times to conduct an inspection as necessary to assure the department that the HHA is in compliance with the standards of quality set out by the department. This inspection may be part of a routine audit of health care facilities or may be in response to a complaint by someone receiving home health services or by someone on behalf of another individual receiving those services.

The department will conduct an inspection as part of investigating any complaints it may have received. It may do the following:

- conduct an unannounced inspection, including a review of medical and personnel records (such records will generally remain on the premises of the HHA unless the HHA allows the department to remove them);
- conduct an interview with a recipient of home health services, which may be conducted in the recipient's home if the recipient and his or her physician consent;
- interview the physician or other health care practitioners who may be providing other services to the patient; and
- interview other caregivers, including family, friends, and neighbors, who may have information necessary to the investigation.

Q.2:11 What are the sanctions for violating requirements to obtain a license?

A person who operates a home health agency without first obtaining a license may be liable for civil monetary penalties, usually a specified amount for each day the person is in violation. In addition, the state may provide for a court to grant irjunctive relief, depending upon the nature and severity of the violation. If an injunction is granted, the HHA would cease operations pending an investigation. [See TAC Title 2, Health, Chap. 142.013-014.]

CERTIFICATE OF NEED FOR HOME HEALTH AGENCIES

Q.2:12 What is a certificate of need (CON)?

A CON is a formal acknowledgment by a state government that a particular health care service or program meets the identified needs of the state in providing health care to its population.

Q.2:13 What is the purpose of requiring health care providers to obtain a CON?

The primary purpose of requiring CONs is to apply the results of the "health planning" process to ensure adequate availability of health care services. During a health planning process, a state assesses the needs of its population and identifies the resources available to meet those needs. The health planning process allows the state to provide health care services in an orderly, planned fashion, and to avoid creating imbalances in the availability of services in the state.

A state will allocate its health care resources based on the need for certain types of services in given geographic areas. For example, the state may determine that a certain suburban area with a younger, healthier population is saturated with home health services, while an older urban area populated disproportionately by elderly persons cannot get access to enough home health services. A home health agency trying to serve the suburban area will be denied a CON, while an agency intending to locate in the urban area will receive a CON.

Q.2:14 How did the CON program develop?

The CON program began at the state level in the late 1960s and was dominated by local and regional health planning entities known then as health systems agencies. In the early 1970s, the federal government entered the arena, providing funding for capital expenditure reviews at the state and local level. Subsequently, funding was available under the Public Health Services Act for states enacting CON legislation that mirrored federal requirements.

The federal scheme was very specific as to the process. It required that states

- observe review cycles that included time limits and batching applications for similar services;
- adhere to notice requirements;
- hold public hearings and compile written findings and conclusions; and

- hold administrative and judicial review proceedings for providers and affected members of the public.

Finally, in the late 1980s, the federal involvement in the CON program diminished, and the states took it over. Some states eliminated the program, but those who have continued it have preserved the features of the federal program. Currently, the statistics regarding home health agencies and other home care providers are as follows:

- Twenty-four states require Medicare-certified agencies to obtain a CON.
- Fourteen states require non–Medicare-certified agencies to obtain a CON.
- Five states require providers of home care (home health aides, personal care aides, homemakers) to obtain a CON.
- Fourteen states require Medicare-certified hospices to obtain a CON.
- Eight states require non–Medicare-certified hospices to obtain a CON.
- Two states require temporary staffing agencies to obtain a CON.
- Four states require providers of IV therapy to obtain a CON.
- One state requires home medical equipment providers to obtain a CON.

[See State Licensure and Certificate of Need Survey, Forum of State Associations, National Association for Home Care, Washington, D.C., February 1994.]

There are great questions about the appropriateness of the CON process. Many states are looking to abolish it, in which case the market will control who operates and who does not operate in a particular state or area within a state. Even when the requirement is universally abolished, the legacy of the CON scheme will remain, as the same criteria used to review applications for CONs and to award them will govern the marketplace. These criteria include the nature of the services, the availability of those services within the geographic area to be served, the nature of the population to be served, and the quality of the services delivered. These criteria are discussed in more detail below.

Q.2:15 What types of entities and services are required to have a CON?

Virtually every state that has the CON process in place requires a CON for hospitals. In addition, many states require CONs for home health agencies, skilled nursing facilities, inpatient rehabilitation facilities, residential care facilities, hospices, kidney disease treatment centers, ambulatory health care facilities, and outpatient clinics.

A very few states require CONs for home IV therapy providers, temporary staffing agencies, and home medical equipment providers. New York categorizes a specific type of agency as a long-term care home health agency, and requires a CON for this type. [N.Y. Pub. Health Law §3610 (McKinney 1985).]

Additionally, a health care facility that intends to incur certain capital expenditures over a specific dollar amount may need to obtain a CON for such expenditures. Finally, most states require a CON for the acquisition of major medical equipment. The definition and dollar value of major medical equipment varies from state to state.

Q.2:16 How long does a CON last?

Once a CON has been granted, the entity must begin the project within a specified period of time. This period could be any amount of time. For example, in California a CON expires 18 months from the date of issuance. If the project is not completed by this time, the office of health planning may extend the completion period for up to 12 months beyond the expiration date if the HHA is diligently pursuing the project to completion or can show good cause why it is not completed.

Q.2:17 In what situations is an entity required to have a CON?

There are several main types of situations in which a CON is required. These range from the construction of new facilities to the addition of new services. More specifically, a CON may be needed in the following circumstances:

- The construction, development, acquisition, or other establishment of a new health care facility or service.
- The partial or total closure of a health care facility or cessation of provision of a health care service. Thus, if a hospital that operates an HHA closes and the HHA ceases operations, the hospital would need to get approval from the health planning board.
- The incurring of any obligation for a capital expenditure by or on behalf of a health care facility or for purposes of providing a health care service.
- The addition of health services that were not offered on a regular basis prior to the time the services are proposed to be offered.
- A substantial change to the number and nature of health care services offered by or on behalf of a health care facility if the change is associated with a previous service for which a CON was issued. Some states provide a time limit on this criterion, so that if the change occurs within, say, two years after the CON was issued, the facility need not obtain a new CON simply for the change. Many states, however, require the new CON for any substantial change, no matter when it occurs. They view the CON requirement very narrowly; if the CON was issued for certain services, it is no longer valid if the services change.
- If the entity operating the health care services sells or leases the facility from which the services are provided. Some states require the CON only if there is substantial change in the services or the geographic area or population to be served. For example, if the HHA formerly served mostly Medicare patients and the new owners or lessees decided to serve primarily pediatric patients, the facility would most likely need a new CON.

In a recent case, a private duty nursing service, which also functioned as a nursing pool, questioned whether it could send nurses
into patients' homes without obtaining a CON. State law exempted
private duty nursing pools from the CON requirement where employees were being sent into health care facilities. The reviewing
court decided that sending nurses into patients' homes was not
within the scope of the exemption, because when nurses were sent
into health care facilities, there were adequate numbers of facility
personnel available to oversee the actions of the nursing pool
personnel. In the home setting, there was no such supervision. If the
nursing pool sent personnel into the home setting, it would be
functioning as a home health agency and thus should be required to
obtain a CON. [*Medical Personnel Pool of Louisville, Inc., v. Management Registry, Inc.*, Nos. 92-CA-000924-MR, 92-CA-000967-MR, Ken-
tucky Court of Appeals, 41 K. L. S. 2, March 3, 1994.]

Q.2:18 If an HHA has either just a license or just a CON, must it obtain the other?

It depends upon the state. Some states use licensure as a prerequisite to issuing a CON, some use CON as a prerequisite to licensure.
In still others, the two are entirely independent.

Q.2:19 What regulatory body issues CONs?

The state department of health planning issues CONs. This division may also be called the "health resources division" or the "state
health planning and development agency." In some cases, the
overall state planning agency is responsible for health planning and
issues CONs.

Q.2:20 How does the CON process begin?

Generally, the process begins in one of two ways. The regulatory
body may issue a notice in the state register of proposed regulations.
This notice will inform the public, including prospective health care
providers, that a specific need exists in the state at that time.

Providers will be encouraged to apply for a CON to furnish services that meet the need.

A prospective applicant may also initiate the process. The applicant will meet with the state planning agency to discuss the state plan and demonstrate how the applicant's proposed new facility or expansion of an existing facility or service is consistent with the plan and will benefit the state. Often the applicant will need to show that the plan is out of date and that the proposed project will bring it up to date.

Q.2:21 What steps are involved in obtaining a CON?

Although the specific process varies from state to state, the basic process is the same for all states that have CON requirements for HHAs. Some states have a specific form that an HHA must use to complete an application, whereas others simply have specific information that must be provided in any format the HHA desires to use.

The HHA pays a fee for filing the application. The fee, which ranges from $1,000 up to $10,000, is set annually by regulation and is different for each type of project and cost of the project.

Before filing the application for a CON, the HHA must notify the health planning office of its intent to apply for the CON. If such notice is not given, the office may refuse to accept the application, but once the CON is issued, the office may not invalidate it solely because the HHA did not give proper notice.

Q.2:22 What information must an HHA provide in a CON application?

The application must contain at least the following information:

- the site of the facility in the geographic area to be served (for an HHA, this requirement is presumably intended for the office quarters of the agency and for the main and branch office if such branches exist);

- the population to be served, as well as the projected growth of that population, described in terms of age, income, and gender;
- the anticipated demand for the health care services to be provided;
- a description of the services to be provided;
- a description of the existing programs within the area to be served offering the same or similar health care services, with an analysis of the utilization of those programs;
- the benefit to the community that will result from the development of the project as well as the anticipated impact on other institutions offering the same or similar services in the area;
- a schedule for the commencement and completion of the project; and
- reasonable assurance that adequate financing is available for the completion of the project within the time period stated in the application.

Q.2:23 What does the health planning office do with an application once it is filed?

The office of health planning reviews the application for completeness. If the application is found to be incomplete (e.g., it does not discuss the above-mentioned topics adequately), the office will notify the HHA to submit the required additional information. After receipt of the additional information, the office will determine whether the application is complete within a specific period of time. This time is usually fairly short, possibly only 30 days. Maryland, however, has up to 150 days to act on the application, and New Jersey has no time limit, as it acts on applications that are similar in a group fashion. The planning office may not request any information outside the scope of its original request.

If upon a subsequent completeness review the application is still found to be incomplete, the HHA may either submit the additional information required by the office or request in writing that the full CON review be undertaken. Unless the omission is so material that it would cause any substantive review to be meaningless, the review will commence.

During review, the application may be amended or withdrawn by the HHA at any time "without prejudice." This means that the HHA would not be prevented from further amending the application or, if it is withdrawn, from filing another application at a later date simply because the HHA withdrew an application at this particular time. The term indicates that "no rights or privileges of the party concerned are to be considered as thereby waived or lost except in so far as may be expressly conceded or decided." [*Black's Law Dictionary*, 5th ed., West Publishing Co., 1979.] Thus, as long as the HHA did not expressly indicate that it would never file another application, it may, indeed, do so at any later time.

The filed application is a matter of public record and is available for inspection at the health planning office. Most states involve the public through the announcement of hearings and through delegating local health planning agencies to comment on the applications.

Q.2:24 What process does the health planning office follow in considering a filed application?

Within 30 days or so of receipt of the complete application, the office of health planning does one of two things. It can approve the application, possibly modifying or adding conditions that the HHA must agree to in writing. If the office determines that "substantial" questions exist as to the appropriateness of the proposed project, it will order a hearing to be held in the health service area proposed to be served by the HHA.

The hearing notice will be published in at least one newspaper of general circulation in the health service area to give the public an opportunity to express views on the necessity of the services that the HHA intends to provide. The hearing will begin shortly after the date the office orders the hearing and will be limited in time. This time period may be extended if the HHA agrees to extend it or if the hearing continues during consecutive business days beyond the expected date of conclusion.

Within a short period of time, possibly as short as only seven days, after the conclusion of the hearing, the hearing officer will issue a proposed decision that will be sent to all parties. The director of the health planning office will issue a final decision on the application soon after the hearing officer issues the proposed decision. The final decision will be published in a newspaper of general circulation within the health service area served by the HHA within ten calendar days following the decision.

The final decision will either approve the application (with or without modifications), reject it, or approve it with conditions mutually agreed upon by the office and the HHA. The CON may be revoked if the HHA does not fulfill the conditions under which it was granted.

Q.2:25 Wha⸱ criteria does the health planning office use to evaluate an application?

The federal program enumerated specific criteria for evaluating applications. These criteria were adopted, if not directly, then indirectly by the state programs after the demise of the federal program. The criteria include

- the relationship between the proposed health service and the state health plan;
- the availability of less costly alternatives;
- the need of the population for the proposed services in the area serviced by the provider;
- the extent to which the proposed services are already being provided in the area;
- the availability of resources to provide the services, including clinical and management personnel, funding for the services, and ancillary and support services;
- the competitive effect of the addition of the services to the area;
- the fostering of cost containment;

- the level of service and the quality of care provided by the provider in delivering its existing services.

Q.2:26 What are an HHA's options if a CON is denied?

The HHA may file an appeal if it has appropriate grounds.

Q.2:27 What are the procedures for appealing the denial of a CON?

The HHA may appeal the denial of a CON if it has appropriate grounds. These grounds include the following:

- The health planning office or hearing officer, if a hearing was held, violated the procedures.
- The decision of the office or hearing officer is not supported by substantial evidence.
- The office or hearing officer acted arbitrarily or capriciously.

The appeal procedures are similar to procedures for filing the CON application, with public notice in a newspaper of general circulation and fairly stringent timelines for each step of the process. The appeals board or council either affirms or reverses the decision and may also remand it to the original decisionmaking body, which means it goes back for review by that body. The second review by that original body will be final. In some states, the HHA may skip the appeal process through the state agency and go directly to the courts.

Q.2:28 What sanctions may be applied if the HHA operates without a CON?

In states where a CON is required in order to operate, the HHA may have its license revoked and will most likely be permanently prohibited from operating in the state (e.g., California and Maryland). In addition, the state may impose a monetary penalty upon the HHA.

In some states where a CON is required, failure to obtain a CON may not result in penalties, except that the HHA will not be able to obtain Medicare reimbursement. In other states, the state agency may have authority to seek injunctive relief to prevent construction of a facility or operation of an HHA in violation of the CON requirement.

3

Business-Related Legal Issues

In addition to obtaining the necessary permits to operate, a home health agency must also decide upon the mode in which it will operate. It must determine its legal structure, based upon the nature of the individuals involved in the business; the financial resources of the business; and the agency's short- and long-term goals. Indeed, the nature of the agency's business may change over time, and the legal structure may also change in response. The key for the home health agency is to consider changes to the legal structure in light of its strategic planning.

The home health agency must consider other legal issues during the course of its existence as a business entity. It may at some point encounter financial problems that may be alleviated by a bankruptcy, and it will almost certainly encounter situations in which its employees, patients, or suppliers are in bankruptcy proceedings. Bankruptcy may be a deliberate action to further the existence of the agency, but it must be used wisely.

Finally, in the course of its dealings, the home health agency must keep abreast of its relationship to other agencies and to the mode in which those agencies respond to the flow of business in their service area. Antitrust issues are becoming more prominent in the health care arena, and agencies must be aware of situations where they or agencies with which they do business may run afoul of the antitrust laws.

FORMS OF LEGAL ORGANIZATION

Q.3:1 What are the different forms of legal organization that could be used by an HHA?

There are many forms of legal organization that an HHA can consider. The most common forms are the partnership, the corporation, and the limited liability company, which is becoming increasingly popular. Other forms are the sole proprietorship and the limited partnership. Which form is ultimately taken depends upon the goals of the HHA, the availability of investors, and the types of owners.

Q.3:2 What is a sole proprietorship?

In a sole proprietorship, one individual is the owner of the HHA (i.e., that individual owns all of the assets of the agency). The HHA is treated as an extension of the owner rather than as a separate entity. Thus, the revenues and, if applicable, the losses incurred by the business accrue to the owner's personal income tax. While this simplifies accounting, the tradeoff is that the owner is solely liable for all of the actions of the HHA—for debts, contractual obligations, and torts.

One advantage of the sole proprietorship is its simplicity. There are no special filings that must be made with the state and no specific requirements for recordkeeping other than those required for tax and other business purposes. The owner is free to conduct the activities of the business in any manner that complies with applicable law and does not have to convene special meetings or maintain special records merely to track business activities. This form of organization, generally uncommon, is occasionally used by professional practitioners such as physicians in the exercise of their professional activities.

Q.3:3 What is a partnership?

A partnership is an association of two or more persons to carry on, as co-owners, a business for profit. [Uniform Partnership Act, §6(1).]

Each partner shares in the profits, as well as the losses, incurred by the business in proportion to his or her percentage or interest in the business. The partnership is treated merely as a conduit and is not subject to taxation as a separate entity. Thus, the gains and losses of the partnership flow through to the individual partners and are reported on their personal income tax returns.

In terms of management of the business, each partner generally has the authority to legally bind the business. Thus, if a partner enters into a contract, all the partners are bound to honor the terms of that contract. A breach by any one partner implicates all the partners. Additionally, each partner generally has the right to participate equally in the management of the business, indeed, will be presumed to have participated in decisions affecting the business. Therefore, all partners are equally liable for the effects of poor decisions.

Like the sole proprietorship, there are no formal filings with the state to establish the existence of a partnership. It is a creature of contract between the partners. In addition, no special records, other than those for taxation and other business reasons, need be kept.

The downside of a partnership arrangement is that each partner is subject to unlimited liability not only for his or her own acts but for the acts of the other partners and the employees of the partnership acting within the scope of their partnership duties or employment respectively. However, the associated risk can be reduced through the purchase of insurance against property damage, employee misconduct, and malpractice.

Another disadvantage of the partnership arrangement is that potential investors may be deterred by the essential factors of its operation: that the partners are actively involved in management and have unlimited liability.

Q.3:4 What is a limited partnership?

A limited partnership will have two types of partners: general partners and limited partners. A limited partner cannot exist without at least one general partner. The general partners function as described above—they participate in and control the management functions of the business and assume unlimited liability. Generally, one or more general partners, whether individuals, corporations, or other entities, must have, for tax purposes, a net worth sufficient to prevent a collapse of the limited partnership. Limited partners, as their name suggests, have limited participation and control but also limited liability. In some respects, a limited partner is viewed as a mere investor in the entity. If, however, at critical times in the life of the business a limited partner is viewed as participating in the management or operations of the business or the limited partnership is undercapitalized, that partner may be construed as a general partner and may therefore be open to unlimited liability.

Q.3:5 What is a corporation?

The most common form of organization is the corporation. This form has advantages that neither the sole proprietorship nor the partnership possesses. In essence, the corporation is a creature of statute, a type of "contract" between the entity and the state as to how the entity will be formed and operated. The laws of a particular state control the scope of the formation of corporate entities in that state, generally through specified requirements for the articles of incorporation or charter that must be filed with the state corporation office.

The corporation is itself a legal entity separate from any of the parties involved in the formation or management of the entity. The owners of the corporation are the stockholders, and they elect a board of directors to formulate policies by which the company is run. These policies are called the bylaws of the corporation. The directors, in turn, appoint officers to run the corporation on a day-to-day basis. Thus, the individual stockholders neither manage the activities of the corporation nor can they legally bind the entity. In fact, other than through their ability to elect directors, the individual stockholders generally can do little to affect how the corporation is run.

Use of the corporate form may make the HHA more attractive to investors. If individuals choose to become involved in the management of the entity, they may do so as officers or directors and will be protected from the liability so threatening in a partnership or sole proprietorship arrangement. In addition, assuming that the stock will grow in value, investors will have a marketable asset, and any gain over a long period will be taxed at a more favorable rate than if treated as individual income.

Q.3:6 What is a limited liability company?

The limited liability company (LLC) is a new form of business organization and is fast becoming a favored legal format for health care entities. Its main advantage is that it provides the owners of a business entity the same protection from liability that the corporate form affords its stockholders while also treating those owners as partners for purposes of federal and state income tax.

Operationally, the LLC most resembles a partnership. The "partners" are refered to as *members*, the term many state statutes use to refer to the owners. In some states, the authority of the members is the same as in a general partnership arrangement. Each member is an agent of the LLC and has the authority to bind the LLC. In contrast to a partnership arrangement, however, in many states the LLC may include a "limitation statement" in its organizing documents that indicates to third parties that the members do not in fact have the authority to bind the LLC. [See, e.g., Md. Code Ann. Corps. and Ass'ns. Article §§4A-101 *et seq.*] While state statutes vary in the scope of the limitations possible for the liability of members, this limitation remains the cornerstone of the LLC concept and ensures that it will continue to be a popular option.

BANKRUPTCY LAW

Q.3:7 What is bankruptcy?

Bankruptcy is a mechanism by which a person or entity that cannot pay the bills that are due obtains relief from the obligation to pay. [*Black's Law Dictionary*, 5th ed., West Publishing Co., 1979.] The person or entity obtaining relief from payments, or debts, is known as the *debtor*, and the person or entity to whom the debt is owed is known as the *creditor*.

Q.3:8 Who can become a debtor?

A debtor can be someone who resides, is domiciled, has a place of business, or has property in the United States. There are certain conditions and requirements for each type of bankruptcy, including, for example, limits on the amount of debt.

Q.3:9 In what capacity might an HHA be involved in a bankruptcy proceeding?

The HHA may be a creditor in a number of situations. First, the HHA may be owed a debt by a patient who files for bankruptcy. Or the HHA may be a creditor of an employee to whom it has advanced salary payments, and who files for bankruptcy before satisfying that debt. Commonly, an employee will file for bankruptcy upon learning that his wages will be garnished to satisfy a judgment against him, and the HHA must comply with the garnishment until it receives notice of the bankruptcy filing. The HHA may be a creditor of a third-party payer by virtue of having provided home health care services to one of the payer's insureds. Finally, it is possible that the HHA will become a debtor in a bankruptcy action, as a means, for example, of buying time until Medicare payments are received.

Q.3:10 What are the types of bankruptcy proceedings an HHA might be involved in?

There are four different types of bankruptcy proceedings provided for in the bankruptcy code. [11 U.S.C. §§101 *et seq.*] These are known as chapters because they are found in certain chapters of the code. They include Chapter 7 (Liquidation), Chapter 11 (Reorganization), Chapter 12 (Family Farmer), and Chapter 13 (Adjustment of Debts of an Individual with a Regular Income) proceedings. The three most common types of bankruptcy proceedings in which an HHA might be involved, either as a creditor or debtor, are Chapter 7, Chapter 11, and Chapter 13 proceedings.

Q.3:11 What is Chapter 7 and in what situations would an HHA benefit from it?

Chapter 7 involves a liquidation of the assets of the debtor. The purpose of a Chapter 7 proceeding is for the debtor to completely discharge all its debts. A trustee is appointed by the bankruptcy court to oversee the liquidation and to ensure that any assets are distributed according to the priorities in the code. Most Chapter 7 debtors have no assets available, particularly for unsecured creditors. Any assets usually fall within the allowed exemptions, such as a portion of equity in a principal residence, part of the value of a motor vehicle, tools and equipment of the debtor's trade, and pension and retirement funds.

An HHA is likely to encounter a Chapter 7 proceeding by a patient or employee. A patient who has filed a Chapter 7 petition will likely have any debt to the HHA discharged. An employee who has filed a Chapter 7 petition may be subject to wage garnishment by the Court, and the HHA will have to ensure that the garnishment is performed.

Q.3:12 What is Chapter 11 and how does it apply to an HHA?

Chapter 11 typically applies to business entities rather than individuals; thus it is the most likely type of proceeding an HHA would use if it were to file for bankruptcy. It is known as a "reorganization," and the goal is to negotiate with creditors regarding what portion of the debts will be repaid and under what terms. Under this chapter, the HHA would continue to maintain its business as a "going concern" rather than liquidate its assets. Thus, the HHA could continue to provide services while reorganizing.

Under this chapter, the debtor, usually a business entity, proposes a repayment plan, which must then be approved by the court. All creditors receive a disclosure statement containing detailed information about the debtor's financial situation. Creditors also receive a copy of the plan and have the opportunity to object if appropriate. Thus, an HHA might be a creditor of a managed care entity or another provider, such as an infusion provider, with which the HHA had an agreement to provide services. If the provider filed for bankruptcy under Chapter 11, the HHA would have an opportunity to approve the provider's repayment plan and continue to operate under the agreement while the plan was being formulated.

Q.3:13 What is Chapter 13 and how does it apply to an HHA?

Chapter 13 is designed for individuals who are wage earners. They commit their disposable income to a repayment plan. "Disposable income" is defined as funds remaining available for commitment after the debtor's reasonable expenses are paid. It is paid to the bankruptcy trustee, who then takes his or her fee and disburses the remaining funds to creditors following the provisions of the plan. In this type of situation, an HHA would be a creditor listed in the plan and receive payments under that plan.

Q.3:14 How does the filing of a bankruptcy petition by a debtor affect an HHA?

The specific answer depends upon the type of bankruptcy. There are, however, some common consequences. The moment bankruptcy is filed, an automatic stay goes into effect. The automatic stay gives the debtor a "fresh start." [11 U.S.C. §362(a); *Perez v. Campbell*, 402 U.S. 637 (1971).] This means that creditors cannot take any action to collect a debt without permission of the court. The statute provides for many exemptions from the automatic stay and for certain grounds on which the court can "lift" the stay if the creditor brings the issue before the court.

If the debt to the HHA is secured by property, relief from the stay will be required for repossession of that property. For example, if the patient has equipment in the home and has not made the payments on that equipment, the HHA would need to get permission from the court to repossess that equipment. If, however, a creditor obtains any type of property from the debtor in violation of the automatic stay, that action will be invalid.

Q.3:15 What if an HHA has a contract with another provider and one of the parties files for bankruptcy protection?

The bankruptcy code specifically addresses the issue of contracts and leases with bankrupts, referring to them as "executory contracts" and "unexpired leases." For example, an HHA may have a contract to provide skilled nursing services to a home infusion provider or a contract to use the services of that home infusion provider for the HHA's patients. An executory contract, therefore, is one in which the duties of at least one of the parties are ongoing and were not fully performed at any one time.

The debtor in the bankruptcy proceeding, which is the party that filed for bankruptcy, has the right to assume or reject the executory contract. In fact, this right may be a primary reason for the choice to file for bankruptcy. The debtor may choose to reject unprofitable contracts merely by showing that the rejection is of benefit to the debtor.

This rejection of an executory contract must be done through the bankruptcy trustee; it cannot be an independent decision by the bankrupt party. If, however, the debtor chooses to assume the contract, the debtor must cure any default (meaning the contract should be brought current) or provide adequate assurance that the trustee will promptly cure any default. [11 U.S.C. §365.]

For example, if an HHA files for bankruptcy, it can elect to continue providing skilled nursing services to the IV therapy provider or it can elect to cease providing those services. If the HHA assumes the contract, the IV therapy provider must honor the contract even though the IV therapy provider may be somewhat skeptical of the HHA's current situation. If the HHA elects to reject the contract, the IV therapy provider cannot enforce it against the HHA. Similarly, the IV therapy provider that has filed for bankruptcy can elect to assume or reject its contract with the HHA, and the HHA may not refuse to perform or compel performance contrary to the decision of the IV therapy provider.

Q.3:16 Must a bankrupt party that has assumed an executory contract personally perform the services under that contract?

No, the bankrupt party may assign the contract or lease to a third party, even if the contract prohibits such assignment. Thus, the HHA could assume a contract and then assign it to another HHA, in which case the second HHA would provide the services. Conversely, however, if the IV therapy provider referred to above decides to assign its contract with the HHA, the HHA may be stuck with the services of an IV therapy provider with which it does not wish to do business.

Q.3:17 What action should an HHA take in response to the filing of a Chapter 13 bankruptcy petition by one of its debtors?

A patient or provider to whom the HHA has furnished services may still owe the HHA for those services at the time of the Chapter 13 filing. The HHA should always review the proposed repayment plan submitted by the debtor. First, the HHA must determine if the debt is secured by collateral, or some kind of property, or is unsecured.

If the debt is secured, the HHA will be paid according to the value of the collateral securing the debt. The HHA should ensure that it is being paid the fair market value of the collateral. It should also request "adequate protection" payments, which ensure that the HHA is paid enough from the very beginning to compensate for the depreciation of the collateral during the life of the plan.

If the debt is unsecured, the HHA should ensure that the plan is providing for all of the debtor's disposable income to be paid to the trustee. The HHA must carefully review the entire plan, not just the parts that relate to the HHA's debt, to ensure that the debtor has not included luxury expenses that lower the amount of the payments the debtor can make. Unsecured creditors receive a certain percentage of their claim, depending upon how much money the debtor pays. The more the debtor pays into the plan, the higher the percentage of the payment to unsecured creditors.

The HHA must always file a proof of claim with the court by the deadline provided in the notice sent to the HHA and all other creditors by the court. Without a claim, the HHA will not even be in the running to receive any percentage of the debtor's payments under the bankruptcy plan. The debtor may contest the HHA's claim by filing an objection with the court, and the judge will decide if the claim is valid.

Q.3:18 What should an HHA do if one of its debtors files a Chapter 11 bankruptcy?

The Chapter 11 debtor must also file a plan with the court but has a longer period of time in which to do so. As with the Chapter 13, the HHA should carefully review the plan to be sure that its debt is provided for. The court will send a notice giving a deadline for filing a claim, but it is advisable to file even before the notice is received.

Q.3:19 How does a Chapter 7 bankruptcy differ from other types of bankruptcy?

A Chapter 7 filing does not commit the debtor to provide any future income for the benefit of creditors. There is no plan, as with the other chapters. If the creditors receive any payment, it comes from the assets that the debtor had before the filing of the petition. In most Chapter 7 filings, the HHA will get no payment. If the debt is secured, the debtor must bring the payments current. If the debtor cannot bring the payments current, the HHA can ask the court to return its collateral.

Q.3:20 What are the consequences of a discharge from debt?

When a bankruptcy is over, the debtor receives a discharge from its debts. [11 U.S.C. §524.] The discharge acts as a prohibition, or injunction, against any collection, recovery, or offset of any debt as a personal liability of the debtor. Once the discharge has occurred, creditors cannot collect debts that were disclosed and dealt with during the bankruptcy, even if no payment was received on those debts. At this point, the automatic stay is lifted, so if the HHA has a secured debt, it can repossess the property without authorization from the court if payments are not being made and kept current.

In one recent case, however, the court would not discharge a patient's debt to an HHA, and the HHA was able to recover sums owed to it because the patient's insurance benefits had been assigned to the HHA. For some reason, the insurance company mailed the benefits to the patient, who chose to spend the money rather than pay the debt to the HHA. The court found that the patient had embezzled the proceeds, which were the property of the HHA under §523(a)(4) of the bankruptcy code, and would not discharge the patient's debt. [*Quality Homecare Services v. Hadley*, No. 93-61260, U.S. Bankruptcy Court for Northern District of N.Y., May 26, 1994.]

Q.3:21 What occurs when an HHA is the debtor in bankruptcy?

If an HHA decides to file for bankruptcy, it will most likely do so under Chapter 11, which is the chapter involving business reorganization. This type of bankruptcy is usually filed to give the HHA time to reorganize its business, eliminate unnecessary debts, and re-establish its financial position. Often it is filed to avoid imminent harm, such as the repossession of equipment or other property necessary to conduct its business.

Numerous pitfalls stand in the way of creditors in the Chapter 11 situation. Sometimes the debtor will delay the filing of the plan and deplete the company's resources, resulting in the conversion of the petition to a Chapter 7, in which case no payment at all is made to creditors. Predictably, the debtor will also make some of the same management mistakes that led to the financial problems in the first place.

Under a Chapter 11, the seven largest creditors may form a creditors' committee. This committee will consult with the debtor, investigate the debtor's financial situation, and participate in the formulation of a plan. Of course, the plan must still be confirmed by the court, but at least the creditors have had an opportunity to protect their interests.

Usually in a Chapter 11, the debtor acts as the trustee and is called the "debtor in possession." Thus the HHA can retain control over its assets and its business operations even as it is reorganizing under the bankruptcy chapter. If, however, a creditor suspects dishonesty or mismanagement by the debtor, the creditor can request that the court appoint a trustee.

Q.3:22 What factors should influence an HHA's decision to file for bankruptcy?

Filing a petition for bankruptcy protection obviously has benefits for the provider, but it may also be detrimental. For example, entities that have been providing the HHA working capital or funds for other purposes may not wish to continue dealing with the HHA. They may try to have the debts owed to them before the petition was filed offset from the payments they are supposed to pay the HHA so that they will not have to continue to pay the HHA any sums during the bankruptcy. This process could affect cash flow to such a degree that business reorganization during the bankruptcy becomes impossible.

In addition, once the HHA has filed for Chapter 11 protection, suppliers will often insist on cash-basis purchases, either in advance, upon delivery, or under extremely short payment terms. Thus the assets must be allocated to maintaining current business before being allocated to pay existing creditors.

Another factor to consider is the effect of the filing upon the HHA's market position. Patients may be reluctant to obtain services from the HHA, as they will perceive that the quality of care will likely suffer due to the economic problems the HHA is experiencing. The HHA's employees may have the same reaction and obtain employment with a competing HHA for fear of losing their jobs or being forced to provide care with fewer resources. Finally, competing HHAs are likely to have a field day with the filing, using it as an opportunity to gain the patients who may choose to leave the HHA. These factors are obviously difficult to adequately evaluate, but they should figure in some way into the HHA's decision about whether or not to file for Chapter 11 protection.

Q.3:23 What is the effect of filing a petition for bankruptcy upon an HHA's payments from the Medicare program?

An intermediary may adjust payments to an HHA if it has a valid belief, based upon reliable evidence, that the HHA has already filed for bankruptcy or will do so shortly or that the HHA may become insolvent. [42 C.F.R. §413.64(i).] In addition, the Medicare program may, in certain limited circumstances, recover overpayments relating to services furnished before the petition was filed from payments relating to services furnished after the bankruptcy has gone into effect. For example, in one case, Medicare suspended payments to an ambulance company that had recently filed under Chapter 11 because Medicare had begun an investigation into whether that company had been overpaid by Medicare. The court found that Medicare's suspension of payments violated the automatic stay because the investigation was not complete and the issue of the overpayment had not been resolved. Therefore, Medicare had to continue paying the company and return any payments it had withheld. [*In re: Medicar Ambulance Company Inc.*, 1994 WL 178850, U. S. Bankruptcy Court for the Northern District of California, May 6, 1994.]

An HHA that has filed a Chapter 7 petition has no right to any periodic interim payments (PIP) in compensation for services furnished after the filing. Under Chapter 7, the HHA will be presumed to have ceased business operations, and Medicare will require return of any periodic interim payments that were made. [See *In re Visiting Nurse Services of Western Pennsylvania*, CCH Medicare and Medicaid Guide ¶37,958 (Bankr. W. D. Pa. 1989).]

Q.3:24 What is the effect of filing a petition for bankruptcy upon the provider agreement?

Prior to 1989, HCFA had the authority to refuse to enter into provider agreements with insolvent or bankrupt providers, but this authority no longer exists.

In addition, some courts have found that the provider agreements are executory contracts and may be assumed or rejected by the debtor. [See *In re: Advanced Professional Home Health Care*, 94 B.R. 95 (E.D. Mich. 1988).] Thus, the HHA could continue as a provider under Medicare but would be required under §365 of the bankruptcy code to cure any valid prepetition claims under the agreement. Other cases, however, have held that the provider agreement is not an executory contract but rather indicates a merely statutory relationship and therefore is not subject to the rules of the bankruptcy code because they apply only to commercial contracts. [See *Lee v. Schweiker*, 739 F.2d 870 (3d Cir. 1984).]

Q.3:25 What is the effect of filing a petition for bankruptcy upon a provider's exclusion from the Medicare or Medicaid program for fraud or abuse?

The bankruptcy code provides for an exception to the automatic stay for governmental actions brought to enforce the government's policy or regulatory powers. This provision prevents use of the bankruptcy process by debtors who improperly seek refuge from their illegal actions. While an exclusion for fraud and abuse clearly qualifies as one of those governmental actions, the crimes causing the exclusion are held to be so serious that a bankrupt provider is not allowed relief under the automatic stay. [See *Chappel v. The Inspector General*, HHS Departmental Appeals Board, Civil Remedies Division, No. C-241, Nov. 8, 1990; *U.S. v. Mickman*, 144 B.R. 259 (E.D. Pa. 1992).]

ANTITRUST LAW

Q.3:26 What is antitrust liability?

The antitrust laws represent an attempt to regulate economic competition so that the playing field is level for all who choose to enter the game. The ultimate question posed by the many different laws and regulations with antitrust content is whether the activity being challenged is primarily procompetitive or anticompetitive.

Q.3:27 What are the main forms of anticompetitive conduct that may violate the antitrust laws?

The most common forms of antitrust violations are the following:

- creating a monopoly through market allocation among competitors;
- agreeing with competitors to fix prices;
- organizing a group boycott or a "concerted refusal to deal" with certain competitors;
- forming an exclusive dealing arrangement; and
- forming a tying arrangement.

Q.3:28 What basic factors are analyzed under antitrust law?

The basic factors in any antitrust analysis are these:

- the market itself;
- the types of activities occurring in that market (activities are categorized as either "horizontal" or "vertical");
- the nature and amount of competition occurring in the market;
- the relationship between the entities in the market;
- the relative strength of providers in the market vis-à-vis other providers in that market (referred to as "market share" or "market power").

Q.3:29 How is the extent of the market determined?

The first step in any antitrust analysis is to identify the market that is to be analyzed. Whether or not anticompetitive activity exists can only be, determined in relation to a given market. Markets are defined by two criteria: the product being provided and the geographic area in which the product is provided.

Product markets are difficult to define because it is hard to know how many different products to include in the market. For example, a general, acute care hospital may be located across the street from a facility that specializes in plastic and reconstructive surgery. The two hospitals may not be competitors, as their products are different and their patients will therefore be different. Thus, the patients will not be adversely affected by any interaction between them that may appear to restrict access to or combine particular services. An HHA specializing in pediatric cases clearly has a different product than an HHA serving primarily elderly persons and would not be a competitor. So, if the two agencies wanted to share pricing information, they could do so without adversely affecting their consumers.

Geographic markets are more straightforward. Generally, the more specialized the service, the larger its geographic market (the area in which most potential customers live). The geographic market for obstetrics and gynecology will likely be relatively small, while the geographic market for neonatal intensive care may be substantially larger. In defining a geographic market, one must consider all the potential competitors in the area. In general, the larger the geographic area included in the market, the lower the market share of any particular provider and the more competition there will be.

Q.3:30 How are horizontal and vertical activities defined and analyzed for purposes of applying antitrust law?

Horizontal activities are the most likely to result in antitrust violations. They are called "horizontal" because they involve a relationship between competitors functioning at the same level in the marketplace, such as between two manufacturers or between two distributors. Assuming two entities have been determined to be competitors, any agreement between them will be suspect. If, for example, two HHAs agree to provide certain services for certain charges (i.e., price fixing), the agreement would be viewed as a horizontal action generally in violation of antitrust laws.

Vertical activities involve players that function at different levels in the marketplace. Such activities might involve manufacturers and distributors, for example, or distributors and retailers. These types of activities are not as suspect because they often result in greater "efficiencies" without negatively affecting competition. The perceived efficiency may serve as a defense to a charge of antitrust violation if the defendant can prove a reduction in costs or prices to consumers or an increase in the quality of the product or service provided.

Q.3:31 What are the two major modes of analyzing antitrust cases?

The two major theories of analysis are the "rule of reason" and the "per se" method. The rule of reason applies in the majority of antitrust cases. It requires a review and an analysis of the "big picture," including the market in which the defendant operates. The object is to consider all of the facts and determine whether they indicate the furthering of competition or the stifling of competition.

Many specific types of activities, on the other hand, have been determined to always restrict competition, by increasing prices, decreasing output, or both. These types are referred to as *per se* violations, and they are presumed to be anticompetitive in that they are inherently unreasonable. Examples include both horizontal and vertical price fixing, horizontal division of markets, concerted refusals to deal ("boycotts"), and tying arrangements.

Historically, transactions involving health care professionals and their services were rarely subject to antitrust review. Such transactions were not suspect because they involved the "learned professions" (and therefore were not "commerce" as defined in the Sherman Act), and because the motivation was not primarily economic but more concerned with quality of care. Recent cases, however, have clearly treated conduct on the part of health care professionals that is truly anticompetitive in the same manner as conduct not related to the learned professions or to health care. [See *Goldfarb v. Virginia State Bar*, 421 U.S. 773 (1975); *Arizona v. Maricopa County Medical Society*, 457 U.S. 332 (1982).]

Q.3:32 How are the nature and amount of competition occurring in the market determined?

These factors are measured by the amount of the difference in price that must exist before a consumer will turn to another provider for the services. For example, if two shoe stores are located a block away from each other, it is likely that if one store raises its prices by 1 percent, a significant number of customers will switch their business to the store that has maintained the lower price. If, however, the stores were located in neighboring towns, the price differential would have to be much greater to induce customers to patronize the other store. The threshold question would indeed be the market question of whether the stores, since they are located in neighboring towns as opposed to adjacent blocks, are even competitors.

This method of measuring competition is difficult to apply to the health care field for several reasons. Health care services, unlike products such as shoes, are not duplicated, and price may not be the determining factor in a consumer's decision to purchase from another provider. The question of quality may play a more important role in a decision to purchase health care services than it does in a decision regarding clothing or automobiles. In addition, many of the choices that were once the consumer's to make have been taken out of the consumer's hands. With the advent of managed care and the various types of networks, the consumer has limited ability to choose his or her own provider. Thus, any choice of one provider over another may not accurately reflect the desire of the consumer to get good value for money spent.

Q.3:33 How are the relationships between the entities in the market analyzed?

Analysis of these relationships measures whether a suspect activity is undertaken by a single economic entity, in which case there are no antitrust issues, or several economic entities, in which case the problems of antitrust may arise. For example, if two HHAs share some employees, refer patients to one another, and share the cost of a billing service and office supplies, but each tracks and bills its own patients, obtained its own CON, and keeps its profits and losses, most likely these two HHAs would be viewed as two separate entities. They would be barred under antitrust analysis from discussing their charges and agreeing on a common charge (fixing prices) for their services. If, however, the two HHAs merge into one corporation, even if they maintain two branch offices, and they run the branches jointly, even if differently, they may be regarded as integrated and could agree on the charges for their services.

Q.3:34 How is the market share (or market power) of the providers in a given market treated in an antitrust analysis?

The greater a provider's market power, the greater chance of an antitrust violation. The actions by a company with greater market power would generally have a greater effect on the level of competition in that market as a whole.

Q.3:35 What federal laws govern antitrust analysis?

Several federal laws address the different theories of antitrust. Section 1 of the Sherman Act prohibits contracts, combinations, and conspiracies in restraint of trade. [15 U.S.C. §1.] Section 2 of the Sherman Act prohibits monopolization, including attempts and conspiracies to monopolize. [15 U.S.C. §2.]

Section 7 of the Clayton Act prohibits mergers, joint ventures, or acquisitions if they substantially lessen competition or tend to result in a monopoly. [15 U.S.C. §18.] Section 2 of the Clayton Act (known as the Robinson Patman Act) prohibits discrimination in price between different purchasers of particular commodities if that discrimination may substantially lessen competition. [15 U.S.C. §13.] Finally, Section 5 of the Federal Trade Commission Act, which governs trade practices in general, addresses antitrust in particular with its prohibition on unfair methods of competition. [15 U.S.C. §45.]

Q.3:36 What agencies enforce antitrust law?

The Federal Trade Commission and the Department of Justice, Antitrust Division, enforce the federal antitrust laws. In addition, each state has a division of the attorney general's office that specializes in antitrust enforcement of the state's laws.

Q.3:37 How are arrangements between different types of health care providers viewed under antitrust law?

The Federal Trade Commission (FTC) and the Department of Justice (DOJ) recently provided specific guidance for health care providers. The agencies issued policy statements specifically addressing potential antitrust enforcement for the various types of arrangements that may occur between and among hospitals and health care providers. [*See Statements of Enforcement Policy and Analytical Principles Relating to Health Care and Antitrust*, September 27, 1994.]

The statements outline "antitrust safety zones," giving specific circumstances where the federal agencies will not challenge a practice under the antitrust laws unless specific circumstances exist. The policy statements also explain how the FTC and DOJ will analyze business practices that do not fall into these safety zones and specify how such practices can be structured to avoid serious antitrust problems.

Q.3:38 What is the significance of the antitrust statements?

The FTC and DOJ have issued these statements because they believe that the health care industry is deliberately avoiding arrangements and systems that might lead to more efficient provision of health care simply because providers are afraid of being in violation of the antitrust laws. The statements are fairly conservative and do not alter current interpretation of antitrust law. Rather, they apply that body of law to the health care industry in very specific ways. In reviewing the actions of health care providers, the agencies will ultimately continue to use the basic antitrust test: do the practices result in significantly lessened competition which adversely affects the consumers of the products and services?

Q.3:39 What are the nine antitrust statements?

The nine policy statements address the following situations:

Statement 1: Mergers among hospitals;
Statement 2: Hospital joint ventures involving high-technology or other expensive medical equipment;
Statement 3: Hospital joint ventures involving specialized clinical or other expensive health care services;
Statement 4: Providers' collective provision of non–fee-related information to purchasers of health care services;
Statement 5: Providers' collective provision of fee-related information to purchasers;
Statement 6: Provider participation in exchanges of price and cost information;
Statement 7: Joint purchasing arrangements among health care providers;
Statement 8: Physician network joint ventures; and
Statement 9: Analytical principles relating to multiprovider networks.

While none of the statements directly addresses home health issues, they affect HHAs because of their involvement in the developing networks of providers and other changes sweeping through the health care system. For example, an HHA may be involved in a hospital merger if the HHA is either owned and operated by the hospital or contracts with the hospital to provide HHA services. Or an HHA may participate in a joint venture with physicians to provide HHA services to patients treated by the physicians. A discussion of each safety zone or principle follows.

1. **Mergers among hospitals**. Most of the hospital mergers do not violate antitrust laws because the hospitals are not significant competitors of each other. Even when a merger reduced the number of competing hospitals in an area to a point which could potentially cause antitrust problems, the agencies have not pursued any action where impressive cost savings have resulted.

The agencies will not challenge the merger of two hospitals if at least one of them has fewer than 100 licensed beds, an average daily census of fewer than 40 patients, and is more than 5 years old. The agency will examine whether the merger allows the resulting entity to exercise undue influence on the cost of hospital services, whether the cost savings are significant enough to look the other way in the antitrust analysis, and whether the hospital that was absorbed was probably not going to survive even without the merger.

2. **Hospital joint ventures involving high-technology or other expensive medical equipment**. The policy statement allows for joint ventures between hospitals to purchase high-technology or other expensive equipment if the shared purchase results in savings for the hospitals. As long as the venture does not include any hospital other than those necessary to create the intended cost savings and does not include any hospitals that could have competed with the hospital in offering that service, the agencies will not challenge the venture.

3. **Hospital joint ventures involving specialized clinical or other expensive health care services**. While not providing a safety zone, the agencies stress that the development of joint ventures between hospitals for the purpose of providing certain services does not necessarily violate antitrust laws. As an example, the statement prohibits two hospitals that both profitably provide services such as a burn unit and open heart surgery unit from simply agreeing, in the absence of an "integrated joint venture," to offer the services at only one of the hospitals. To do so would be an illegal market allocation. The agencies would look at the competitive effect of a venture and evaluate collateral agreements that may unreasonably restrict competition without contributing to the legitimate purpose of the venture. The statement gives the example of a venture to provide oncology services, with a collateral agreement relating to radiation therapy services which may also be provided to nononcology patients. Thus, the collateral radiation therapy services would be

unnecessary to achieve the benefits of the oncology joint venture and would be questioned, while the oncology joint venture itself would be legal.

4. **Providers' collective provision of non–fee-related information to purchasers of health care services.** Providers of all types may collectively provide certain types of information to purchasers of health care services. They may provide information such as medical data and practice parameters that are related to the standards for patient management. They may not, however, collectively boycott or threaten to boycott any purchaser because they object to the purchaser's administrative, clinical, or other terms and conditions governing the provision of services or because the purchaser chooses not to utilize their information.

5. **Providers' collective provision of fee-related information to purchasers.** Providers may provide fee-related information to purchasers of their services as long as they meet certain specified conditions. The collection of data must be managed by a third party, must include information more than three months old, and the information must be based on data from at least five hospitals and aggregated so that the data from particular hospitals cannot be identified. The providers may not boycott or threaten to boycott to coerce purchasers to accept their collectively determined fees. Finally, they may not provide prospective fee-related information.

6. **Provider participation in exchanges of price and cost information.** Providers may participate in written surveys of prices for services or wages, salaries, or benefits of provider personnel. In order to fall within the safety zone, the survey must be managed by a third party, it must include information more than three months old, and the information must be based on data from at least five hospitals and aggregated so that the data from particular hospitals cannot be identified.

7. **Joint purchasing arrangements among health care providers.** Because joint purchases usually result in such dramatic cost savings for consumers, most such arrangements are not challenged. Such joint purchases

include such goods and services as laundry or food services, computer or data processing services, and prescription drugs and other pharmaceuticals, among other things. The statement specifically protects a joint purchasing arrangement as long as it amounts to less than 35 percent of the relevant product or service and the cost is less than 20 percent of the total revenues from all products or services sold by each participant in the arrangement. Participants in arrangements that do not meet these criteria should not be required to use the arrangement but can be asked to commit to purchase a minimum amount to receive the benefit of the volume discount.

8. **Physician network joint ventures**. The agencies will support networks comprised of physicians in each physician speciality with active hospital staff privileges, if those networks are controlled by physicians and jointly market the services of their member physicians. Such arrangements can provide quality services at reduced costs and may be ultimately procompetitive. The statement distinguishes between exclusive and nonexclusive provider networks. In both types of networks, however, the members participating in the venture or network must share the financial risk associated with the venture. This requirement will ensure that the venture is not merely a sham behind which the participants can hide, and enabling them to work together to fix prices. If they share the financial risk, any price-fixing activities would work to their detriment.

Exclusive networks may comprise only 20 percent or less of the physicians in the relevant geographic market, which will ensure that the venture will not create a monopoly enabling the participants to charge excessively high prices. Nonexclusive networks may comprise up to 30 percent of the providers in the relevant geographic market. Special scrutiny will be given to nonexclusive networks to determine that they are, in fact, nonexclusive and not merely portrayed as such contractually.

As with all of the safety zones, this one is available to joint venturers as a protection against antitrust scrutiny by the

FTC and DOJ. Ventures outside the safety zones may also be legally sound, but they do not have the automatic protection of the safety zone, and the agencies have enumerated the criteria that will be used to evaluate such arrangements. The agencies will analyze the relevant markets to determine if monopoly power is created and will examine the structure and operation of the venture to see if such monopoly potential is a danger.

In addition, the agencies will survey the venture's competitors, including potential competitors, to determine if these entities will be able to continue to provide adequate competition. The agencies will evaluate whether the venture produces efficiencies that will balance out any anticompetitive effect and will review any restraints on services unrelated to the venture. Such additional restraints, for example, on services totally unrelated to the venture would clearly not fall into the safety zone, would not produce efficiencies as a result of the venture, and would, therefore, violate antitrust laws.

9. **Analytical principles relating to multiprovider networks**. The agencies acknowledge the need for guidance as affiliations between otherwise competing providers arise. Because the development of networks is a relatively new phenomenon, the agencies did not go so far as to create an explicit safety zone, but rather addressed some of the issues which may arise in the formation of the networks. Basically, the agencies will determine whether competitors are sufficiently integrated throughout the network so that their agreements on prices or other terms of competition do not amount to unlawful price setting or market allocation. Agreements that provide for substantial risk-sharing among the providers in a network would be evidence of sufficient integration to pass the antitrust.

Even where providers do not agree on prices and furnish information to and receive information from purchasers through a third party, or "messenger," the agreement can be legal. As long as the individual providers in a network have the option to accept or reject relationships with such purchasers independently from the other providers in the network, the network will probably not violate antitrust laws. The agencies will rely upon all of the traditional indicators in analyzing the network, including the market area served, the horizontal and vertical competitive effects, the resulting efficiencies, and the effect of exclusion of particular providers. They also stress that in analyzing the network, they will obtain information not only from providers but also from purchasers and consumers. Specifically, the agencies will likely give substantial weight to information from purchasers who have attempted to switch between providers to avoid a price increase to determine whether providers are still able to compete effectively.

Q.3:40 How can health care entities determine whether contemplated actions may violate antitrust laws?

The FTC and the DOJ provide an opportunity for the entity to obtain review of the proposed venture or arrangement. The FTC will render an "advisory opinion," and the DOJ will perform an "expedited business review." These reviews are nonbinding, but they do offer valuable guidance. The agencies will respond within 90 days after all necessary information is submitted, except for multiprovider networks formed using the guidance in Statement 9, in which case the response time will be 120 days.

Q.3:41 Have there been any cases involving home care and antitrust violations?

The most well-known case of interest to providers of home care in the antitrust area is known as the *Venice* case, after the hospital involved in the case. [See *Key Enterprises of Delaware, Inc. v. Venice Hospital*, 919 F.2d 1550 (11th Cir. 1990), reh'g granted, opinion vacated, 979 F.2d 806 (11th Cir. 1992).] In this case, Venice Hospital ("Hospital"), a hospital with a dominant market share in its geographic area, entered into a joint venture with a local HME supplier ("Supplier") to provide HME services to patients from the hospital.

Another local supplier, Venice Convalescent Aids Medical Supply ("Plaintiff") sued the Hospital because it believed that the Hospital illegally referred all of the Hospital's patients to the Supplier. In antitrust language, the Plaintiff charged that the Hospital unreasonably restricted competition in the area because it pressured HHA nurses to refer HME business to the Supplier in violation of Section 1 of the Sherman Act. In addition, the Plaintiff charged that the Hospital monopolized, or at least attempted to monopolize, the HME market in violation of Section 2 of the Sherman Act.

The Plaintiff won a jury verdict at the trial level, but the court later determined that the Hospital had not violated the antitrust laws. Rather, the Hospital had simply engaged in acceptable marketing practices, and the mere fact that these marketing efforts were effective and indeed highly profitable did not mean that they violated antitrust laws. The practices that the Plaintiff objected to involved the active involvement of Supplier personnel in the decisionmaking process for ordering HME. These activities included the following:

- A Supplier employee was the "patient equipment coordinator" in the discharge planning department of the Hospital and was thus viewed as a member of the Hospital staff. He had exclusive access to patients getting ready to leave the Hospital and to home health agency nurses who would be caring for those patients after discharge. Before he came to work at the Hospital, no HME vendor had ever been allowed to enter the Hospital to solicit business from either nurses or patients.

- The Hospital eliminated its previous policy of rotating access to HME suppliers and allowed the Supplier exclusive access to the patients. If the patient or HHA nurses requested another HME supplier, the Supplier's representative would allow this order, but if no other supplier was requested, the Supplier would take the order by "default."

- Although the Hospital no longer used a rotation system for HME suppliers, it continued to use a rotation system for referring patients to home health agencies. The court found no legitimate business reason for running the HME referrals one way and the HHA referrals another way. In addition, some of the HHA nurses testified that they felt coerced to use the

Supplier's services, and even those that did not feel coerced felt it best to use the Supplier's services because they might be booted out of the Hospital and they relied on the access to patients for their own business.

On appeal, the court agreed with the jury that the Hospital had, indeed, violated the antitrust laws because of the practices described above. Due to a procedural technicality involving the court process and the subsequent settlement of the case by the parties, the original decision has little or no value as a legal precedent. It does, however, offer some facts and circumstances that may be viewed as instructional to an analysis of practices of HME companies and, by extension, other home health providers for antitrust purposes.

First, if an HHA enters into exclusive arrangements with other providers of health care that are in a position to refer business to the HHA, including hospitals and HME suppliers, it must be careful to honor the choice of patients. That is, the agreement should specify that the HHA will not pressure any patient to use any particular service but will let the patient choose his or her provider. The HHA may want to go so far as to offer the patient a choice from several named providers of a particular service.

Agencies should also examine the operating procedures of any party to an agreement. For example, if an HHA enters into an agreement with a hospital, the HHA must make sure that the hospital does not refer exclusively to the HHA or pressure either its discharge planning staff or patients to choose the HHA as the provider of postdischarge home health nursing services. If, on the other hand, the HHA has the patient first and is a party to an agreement with an HME supplier, the HHA must ensure that it allows the patient or discharge planner to choose the HME supplier rather than requiring a particular supplier.

Q.3:42 Are there any guidelines as to the percentage of market share of the home care market that may trigger antitrust scrutiny?

In another set of cases, two HME suppliers and the physician investors in those suppliers have been the focus of antitrust scrutiny by the FTC. The FTC alleged that the parties performed "unfair acts and practices and unfair methods of competition," with the result that the joint ventures created "barriers to entry" by other HME companies and therefore stifled competition in the market. As a result of the investigation, the FTC and the parties have entered into proposed consent decrees, one type of settlement that does not involve going to court. [*Homecare Oxygen and Medical Equipment Co., et al., Home Oxygen and Medical Equipment Co., et al., and Certain Home Oxygen Pulmonologists*; Proposed Consent Agreements with Analyses to Aid Public Comment, 58 Fed. Reg. 60653 (November 17, 1993).]

The two companies offered the pulmonologists the opportunity to become partners, either general or limited, in the companies. An offer of this type is not inherently prohibited, but in this case the companies offered the partnerships to 60 percent of the pulmonologists in each geographic area in which the companies compete. In addition, the pulmonologists in question were among the most prominent in the area and had strong ties to the respiratory therapy departments at local hospitals.

In the FTC's view, patients rarely have a preference for an oxygen supplier, as they have little understanding of oxygen treatment. Also, oxygen for medical use may be prescribed only pursuant to the order of a physician. These two factors lead most patients to rely almost exclusively on the recommendation of their physicians in the choice of an oxygen vendor. In this case, the doctors clearly had an incentive to refer the patients to the companies in which they were financial investors, and as a result of these referrals the companies eventually gained market shares of approximately 60 percent.

As a means of settlement, the doctors agreed that within eight months as many of the doctors as necessary will divest their ownership interests in the companies to achieve the result that no greater than 25 percent of the pulmonologists practicing in the relevant geographic market are affiliated with the companies. In addition, for the next ten years, none of the doctors shall have any ownership interest in any entity engaged in the sale, rental, or lease of oxygen systems in the relevant geographic market if that ownership interest would cause more than 25 percent of the pulmonologists practicing in the area to be affiliated with the entity. The FTC allowed an affiliation rate of 25 percent so that any quality of care benefits from the involvement of the doctors could be maintained. The significance of the 25 percent figure is unclear, and the FTC explicitly said that it did not intend to force the pulmonologists to pull out completely but intended to "diffuse" their power in the oxygen market.

4

Contracting for Services

In developing its strategy for delivering home health services, a home health agency will certainly consider the feasibility of working with other entities to deliver services it cannot deliver as efficiently or effectively. The agency should always have a contractual relationship with each entity, as a contract or agreement allows the parties to go through the negotiation process and delineate in detail the duties and obligations of both. This process minimizes misunderstandings and sets out procedures to remedy such misunderstandings, should they occur.

There are many situations in which an HHA may enter agreements with other entities for services. An HHA may wish to provide services through subcontractors for patient care purposes. For example, the HHA may need to respond to its patients' needs for home medical equipment or intravenous therapy. In addition, these other types of providers may need home nursing services, and thus the companies could enter into one contract for mutually provided services or separate contracts, with each party meeting the other party's needs as appropriate.

In addition, the HHA will need to enter into agreements to obtain the services it needs to run its business, including perhaps contracts with medical supply and pharmaceutical companies, as well as contracts with suppliers of computer, laundry, payroll, and other support services. Contracts for nonmedical services would not contain specific provisions addressing quality of care, patient selection, case management, and other patient care–related issues, but they should otherwise be similar to contracts with health care providers, outlining duties of each party, terms of payment, and other standard contract issues, as described below.

Finally, with the increased effect of managed care arrangements on the manner in which home health agencies provide their care, the HHA will need to understand the mechanics of contracting with managed care entities and how the process differs from traditional contracting.

CONTRACTING FOR ANCILLARY SERVICES

Q.4:1 What elements should be included in an agreement with another provider for services?

The HHA and the entity with which it arranges to obtain services should enter into an agreement, or a contract, addressing the numerous issues that arise in delivering those services. The agreement should, at a minimum, address the following:

- the obligations of the HHA;
- the obligations of the provider of the services;
- provisions for renewal and termination of the agreement;
- a schedule of charges for the services to be provided;
- billing arrangements;
- insurance requirements;
- the legal relationship between the HHA and the provider of services;
- maintenance of licensure, certification, or accreditation; and
- confidentiality provisions.

Each of these contractual elements is discussed in detail below.

Q.4:2 What are some of the obligations of the HHA and the provider?

The HHA and the provider can determine the general duties and obligations required to provide the services and negotiate which party performs them. The following contains suggestions for each party, but duties can be distributed however is best in the individual situation. In this example, it is assumed that the patient has been obtained through the HHA and that the HHA is seeking to use another provider for certain services. The HHA may just as easily find itself in the position of providing services to patients obtained through the provider, such as when a home IV therapy company needs a nurse to administer treatment (assuming it does not provide its own nursing services). Regardless of who performs the duties, the following should be addressed:

Obligations of the HHA

The HHA will most likely want to retain complete authority for the operation of its business.

Availability of Personnel. The HHA should agree upon how and when it will make its personnel available for the provision of services. Generally the service coverage will be continuous—24 hours a day, seven days a week.

Patient Selection. The HHA should retain complete and sole authority over identification of patients appropriate for home care and should retain complete and sole control over the criteria it uses to make the determination of whether a patient meets those criteria. Only after the HHA determines that the patient is appropriate should the patient be viewed as "accepted" by the HHA. By extension, the HHA is obligated to treat the patient only after it has accepted the patient for such treatment.

Case Management. The HHA should be responsible for patient case management. This function includes establishment and ongoing management of a patient's plan of care, including regular assessment of the patient's condition and ongoing plan of care and revision of the plan of care when appropriate.

As part of the case management process, the HHA should facilitate communication with team members, patients, caregivers, physicians, and third-party payers. The HHA should coordinate patient care conferences in consultation with the provider. It should set the intervals for these conferences, perhaps monthly or bimonthly, depending upon the patient's condition, but it should also include a provision that conferences will occur "as medically necessary."

Quality Assurance. The HHA should retain responsibility for quality assurance activities related to the patients serviced by the provider (and all other of its patients as well). This responsibility includes appropriate and ongoing monitoring of the quality of both the nursing services as well as the services provided by the provider, which should be evaluated according to the HHA's established quality assurance plan. The HHA should have a quality assurance committee empowered under the agreement to take necessary action to maintain compliance with HHA's policies and procedures, the physician orders, and the patient's plan of care.

Records. The HHA should retain control over all patient records, including medical records, in accordance with its policies and procedures and as required by licensing, accrediting, or certifying entities. It should furnish the provider with a copy of medical records as necessary to ensure that the provider can furnish its services appropriately.

Patient Education. The HHA should also oversee any patient education that is delivered to a patient as to how to use the provider's equipment or other products. The provider may actually do the training, but the HHA should verify that the materials and the method of training are adequate. The training should include training for the patient's family members or other caregivers.

Obligations of the Provider

The provider should be obligated to perform all of the services related to its particular business. For example, if the HHA is contracting with an HME supplier, the supplier should provide all of the equipment and training related to that equipment. If the HHA is contracting with an IV therapy provider, the IV provider should provide all of the equipment and pharmaceuticals and related services.

The agreement should specify, however, that the patient retains the ultimate choice as to which provider of these types of services is used. If the patient chooses another provider, the provider that is contracting with the HHA will have no obligation whatsoever to the patient, even though the patient is still being served by the HHA.

Availability of Personnel. The agreement should specify the availability of the provider's services. If 24-hour service is required, this should be specified. If the provider will also be delivering training to the patient and the family and caregivers, this also should be specified. The HHA should, however, retain approval over the methods and materials used in this process.

Training. The agreement should specify the availability of the provider's staff to furnish such training of the HHA's personnel as the provider and HHA deem necessary, including instruction of agency personnel in pertinent aspects of the type of treatment the provider is furnishing. For example, if the provider is furnishing IV therapy, training by the provider would have to cover, at a minimum, potential metabolic and mechanical complications, appropriate use of equipment and supplies, and quality assurance and risk management issues.

Coordination. The provider should be required to supply the HHA with the amount and nature of information the HHA needs to understand the full treatment given the patient. This information would include nursing notes and medical records created by provider personnel.

Quality Assurance and Patient Care Conferences. The provider should designate at least one person to be a member of the HHA's quality assurance committee for the sole purpose of reviewing the care of patients served by the provider. This designated person should attend the regular patient care conferences established by the provider and the HHA.

Case Management. The provider should have the responsibility to coordinate with the HHA regarding their involvement in each case.

Delivery. The HHA should clearly explain the duties of the provider regarding delivery of equipment or supplies to a patient.

Generally, the provider will be responsible for transportation and personal delivery and retrieval of products, supplies, and equipment to the patient.

Maintenance of Licensure and Accreditation. The provider should be obligated to maintain its quality standards so that its state licensure is protected. In addition, if applicable, the provider should be required to maintain its accreditation. Any violations of either the licensing or accreditation provisions or standards must be reported immediately to the HHA.

Q.4:3 How long should the agreement last and what should the parties do when their relationship ends?

Term of the Agreement. The agreement should specify the effective date, usually the date written in on the first page of the agreement or at the signature line. It should specify exactly how long the agreement remains in effect (the typical period is one year). Many agreements provide for "automatic renewal" on the same terms and conditions for additional one-year terms unless either party gives written notice of nonrenewal at least 30 days prior to the expiration of the then existing term.

Termination of the Agreement. The agreement should specify the termination at any time upon occurrence of any of the following:

- written notice by one party to the other 30, 60, or 90 days prior to the scheduled termination of the agreement;
- written notice by the provider to the HHA for cause (as defined below):
    —conduct on the part of the HHA that constitutes a felony under the laws of any state in which it conducts business or the laws of the United States or that results in the suspension or exclusion of the HHA from the Medicare or Medicaid programs;
    —negligence, willful misconduct, or failure to comply with the terms of the agreement by either party where the defaulting party has been given written notice of its defi-

ciencies and has failed to correct such deficiencies within 30 days after receipt of such notice;

- dissolution or bankruptcy of either party;
- revocation of the HHA's certificate of need or suspension or revocation of licensure.

Rights and Duties on Termination. The agreement should specify the rights and duties of each party upon termination of the agreement by either party. These include the following:

- payment of all amounts due either party within 30 days of the effective date of termination of the agreement;
- return of all records to the proper party; and
- continuation of the provision of services to each patient already receiving services under the agreement until such time as either party or the patient determines that such services should no longer be furnished.

Q.4:4 What arrangements should the parties make for payment for products and services furnished under the agreement?

The agreement should contain specific provisions regarding billing and fees, including the responsibilities and procedures of each party. It should include provisions for issuing statements for services rendered under the agreement and the expected time for payment, usually within 30 to 60 days of the statement date. If applicable, the agreement should provide for procedures for billing third-party payers. Finally, the agreement should include, either as part of the body of the contract or as an attachment, a fee schedule for the services to be provided by each party.

Q.4:5 What other provisions should a contract include?

Compliance with Law and Agency Procedures. The HHA should require the provider to be in compliance with all applicable laws and rules and regulations of governmental agencies having jurisdiction over its operations or the provision of services to patients of governmentally regulated third-party payers. In addition, the HHA should insist that all provider personnel deliver services in accordance with the HHA's policies and procedures.

Limitations. Neither party should be construed to be in violation of the agreement if it is prevented from performing its obligations for any reason beyond its control, including, but not limited to, acts of God, the elements, floods, strikes, labor difficulties, and laws, rules, and regulations of federal, state, and local governments.

Insurance. Each party should be obligated to maintain, in full force and effect during the entire term of the agreement, at its own expense and cost, professional liability insurance and comprehensive general liability insurance covering the activities and products contemplated under this agreement in certain minimum amounts to be decided upon at the time the agreement is executed. Each party should be required to present proof of insurance upon request by the other party.

Status of the Parties. The agreement should specify the legal status of the parties. It could specify one of the following:

- that nothing in the agreement shall be deemed or construed to create a partnership, joint venture, or any other relationship between either of the parties with each other; or
- that the parties are entering into an employment relationship between one organization and an individual of the other organization (this is highly unlikely in such a contract for services, but it is possible); or
- that each party shall act as and be deemed to be an independent contractor.

Indemnification. Each party to the agreement should consider agreeing to indemnify and hold the other harmless against any and all claims, damages, expenses, and costs resulting from or arising out of its negligent or intentional acts or omissions under the agreement. The HHA should be careful, however, about agreeing to indemnify others, even where the indemnification is mutual. Most liability policies exclude instances where a party has assumed contractual liability, leaving the HHA responsible for the cost of the indemnification.

Confidentiality. This provision is often taken for granted by contracting parties, yet it is important that it be explicit that *all* information exchanged in carrying out the functions of the agreement must be kept confidential. This requirement applies to information in both written and oral form, even that which may not have been intentionally communicated. Thus the contract should include the following:

- a description of the types of material that are confidential (including all information, conclusions, recommendations, reports, advice, manuals, procedures, whether written or oral, or other documents generated by the provider or HHA related to the agreement);
- an agreement to obtain authorization in writing before disclosing any confidential information (any disclosure should be done only within the limits and to the extent of that authorization); and
- an agreement to return to the other party, upon request, all confidential materials.

Assignment. The agreement should contain a provision protecting both parties against the assignment of the agreement, in part or in whole. If assignment is allowed, the provider could substitute another provider to furnish services to the HHA. The new provider might be a company that the HHA does not want to do business with, so the agreement should prohibit assignment without written consent of both parties. It should be mutually written so that neither party can unilaterally assign. The HHA may, however, feel comfortable with each party having the ability to assign its rights or delegate its duties to an affiliated entity without the necessity of obtaining the HHA's approval.

Access to Records. If the HHA treats Medicare beneficiaries, the agreement must contain the provision allowing Medicare to review the records as a condition of the provider participation.

Discrimination. The agreement should warrant that the parties will comply with the provisions of Title VII of the Civil Rights Act of 1964 and that no person will, on the account of race, color, national origin, ancestry, age, religion, creed, handicap, or disability, be excluded from participation, be denied benefits, or otherwise be subject to discrimination with regard to the provision of any care or service.

General Provisions. The agreement should contain standard legal provisions affecting interpretation of the contract, such as

- a provision indicating which state's law will govern in a dispute;
- a statement to the effect that if a court holds one provision unenforceable, all others will remain in effect;
- an acknowledgment that the agreement constitutes the full embodiment of discussions between the parties and that no oral statements shall be binding; and
- provisions for delivering notice under the contract, such as in the case of termination or breach.

MANAGED CARE CONTRACTING

Q.4:6 What is managed care?

Managed care is a process by which health care organizations manage their resources in order to achieve a balance between unlimited access to those resources and cost-effective provision of such resources. Under managed care systems, providers will be rewarded financially for controlling the services they provide rather than being paid directly based upon the volume of those services. Home health agencies used to payment for each service performed for each patient will have to adjust to new methods of pricing their services and new vehicles for providing those services.

It has been said that the hospital administrator of the past used to walk through the halls bragging that the hospital had 90 percent occupancy. Now that same administrator walks through the halls fearing each occupied bed spells economic ruin. This is an exaggeration, of course, but some sort of control over the way resources are spent will be necessary in the years to come. In the managed care arena, HHAs and their patients are no longer the only parties with control over treatment. They will have to learn to deal with third-party payers which have, as their primary interest, the goal of controlling costs.

Q.4:7 What are the main types of managed care entities?

Managed care entities come in many forms, but the major models are the preferred provider organization (PPO), the health maintenance organization (HMO), and the case management organization.

The PPO is a "network" of providers, sometimes including home health agencies, that contracts with an insurer to provide its particular health care services to the insured individuals at a negotiated and presumably discounted rate. The providers gain in volume what they lose in reimbursement for services provided to any one patient.

With an HMO model, individuals pay a regular amount, usually on a monthly basis, to receive most or all of the health care services they need. The providers, on the other hand, receive a predetermined rate per enrollee regardless of the actual services they provide in any given month. This method of purchasing health care is known as a capitated payment arrangement, and under a capitated arrangement the incentive to *not* deliver a service is high.

One of the central issues facing providers is access to these patients, and states are beginning to enact laws that guarantee providers the right to participate in networks. These laws are known as "any willing provider" laws, implying that any provider may participate if certain criteria are met.

Case management organizations are independent entities, neither providers nor insurers. Their main functions are to monitor the care given or projected to be given to a patient with a particular condition and propose the most cost-effective methods to provide the necessary care. Case managers act as brokers for health care services and "shop the market" for the provider willing to provide the services at the lowest rate.

An HHA approaching a case manager must be able to present an organized, cost-justified program for treating a patient, and it often finds itself in the position of providing some services at a loss in order to protect future referrals from that case manager. Case management is clearly a productive function in the context of a contract between an HHA and other providers for services, and such a case management provision should be included in all service agreements between the HHA and other providers. The HHA should, however, carefully observe its own quality standards when bidding cases with an independent case manager, who will be focused primarily on the financial characteristics of the services to be provided.

Q.4:8 What should be included in a contract between an HHA and a managed care entity?

Many elements of a traditional contract, as described above in questions 4:1 through 4:5, should be included in a contract with a managed care entity of any kind. Those elements are standard contractual provisions, and represent the essence of an agreement between two parties for the provision of goods or services. Managed care agreements, however, have certain unique provisions and characteristics:

Verification of Coverage and Notification of Participation. The HHA will want to ensure that patients to whom it is about to provide services are actually covered by the managed care entity, which should provide ready access to the necessary information through a hotline or other method. The HHA should also insist that the managed care entity notify its subscribers that the HHA is a participating provider in the network.

Participation in Utilization Review and Quality Assurance Activities. Given that the underlying goal of the managed care entity is to provide cost-effective care, its utilization review activities are likely to be quite sophisticated, and it will typically employ quality assurance methods as well. The standards used in reviewing utilization and quality should be disclosed to the HHA so that it can remain in compliance with them.

Authorization for Specific Services. The HHA should carefully draft the contract so that the managed care entity cannot require it to provide any services other than those agreed upon as covered services. In addition, the HHA should maintain control over how those services are provided, as long as they meet quality standards.

Exclusivity. The HHA should strive to become the exclusive home health provider for the managed care entity, as this will help it gain the volume it needs to offset the rate discounts. The managed care entity, on the other hand, will want to maintain its ability to contract with other providers, so the issue of exclusivity will likely be a subject of intense negotiation.

In arguing for exclusivity, however, the HHA has to consider whether it is willing or able to accept all of the referrals generated by the managed care entity before committing to be the exclusive provider. As a caveat, the HHA must be vigilant regarding possible antitrust violations involved in becoming an exclusive provider.

Geographic Area. The agreement should clearly delineate the geographic area in which the HHA is expected to provide services. A network may cover subscribers across a large area, and the HHA may not be able to service the entire area. In such a case, the HHA will want to clarify with the managed care entity whether or not it is within its contractual rights to subcontract with providers in outlying regions of the area if the providers meet the applicable quality standards of both parties.

Penalties for Late Payment. The HHA is discounting its services to the managed care entity, and thus prompt payment and the cash flow implications of late payment are crucial issues for the HHA. It should, therefore, negotiate a penalty for late payment of claims. The HHA could, for example, require the managed care entity to pay the HHA's regular rates rather than the discounted rates that form the basis of the contract. Ultimately, the HHA should reserve the right to cancel the contract if late payment occurs with some frequency.

Renewal. The HHA might want to consider automatic renewal of the contract to facilitate continuation of the agreement. If such a provision is included, the HHA must ensure that there is a specific provision for renegotiation of rates at time intervals acceptable to the HHA, perhaps even midway through the contract year. Otherwise, the automatic renewal could lock the HHA into an unproductive rate structure for the coming year.

5

Employment Issues

A home health agency's personnel represent its greatest expense, yet are clearly central to the agency's operation. The agency must maximize its human resources and at the same time keep within the laws that have been established to protect the rights of employees. Many legal issues arise when hiring individuals, and the agency must strive to perfect this part of the process, for the cost of hiring and training is so great that a good hire can save the agency a great deal in the long run. Among the first questions an agency must answer is whether or not to retain a staff member as an independent contractor or an employee, and what sort of contractual arrangement should be structured between the parties.

Beginning with the hiring process and continuing throughout the employment relationship, the agency should ensure that its policies as well as its practices are nondiscriminatory. In addition, the agency will undoubtedly face the issue of substance abuse by employees and should develop a policy to address this problem. The agency, because of the new Family and Medical Leave Act, also has obligations regarding employee leaves of absence. Finally, the agency must ensure compliance with wage and hour laws as well as satisfy its duty to provide a safe workplace for employees.

HIRING STAFF

Q.5:1 What sorts of employees are hired by an HHA?

An HHA may need both medical and nonmedical personnel to provide its services. The HHA may need the services of a physician to attend to patients or serve as medical director, or both. In addition, the HHA will use the services of registered nurses (RNs); licensed practical nurses (LPNs); licensed vocational nurses (LVNs); nurse aides or assistants; attendants; and occupational, physical, speech, and respiratory therapists.

The nonmedical personnel that an HHA needs to hire include an administrator and necessary administrative staff, such as clerical and secretarial staff, marketing and sales staff, and financial staff. Nonmedical personnel would also include individuals who provide cleaning, laundry, and other maintenance services.

Q.5:2 What types of hiring issues must an HHA consider?

An HHA must decide whether it wishes to hire individuals as employees or independent contractors. During the interview process, the HHA must be careful to ask appropriate questions so as to ensure compliance with federal and state antidiscrimination laws as well as laws covering employee leaves for medical reasons. Finally, the HHA must carefully investigate all individuals whom it wishes to engage so as to avoid liability for problems those employees might cause.

Q.5:3 What interviewing procedures must HHA personnel follow?

The interviewer must structure the interview so as to get information about the skills, experience, education, and, if applicable, licensure, that are relevant to the job duties. The questions should reflect the job duties as described in the job description, and the interviewer should ask for appropriate documentation to verify that the skill and other requirements are met.

The interviewer must, however, be scrupulous about the types of questions asked at the interview. Any question that could be construed as an attempt to elicit information about a person's race, age, marital status, religion, disability, or child care responsibilities could come back to haunt the HHA if an applicant believes he or she was unlawfully denied employment due to discrimination. Some dos and don'ts of questioning follow:

- *Don't* ask the applicant to provide a photograph with the application (race). *Do* tell the applicant a photograph will be required after hiring.
- *Don't* ask the applicant to indicate what year he or she graduated from school (age). *Do* tell the employee that verification of age may be required after hiring for purposes of compliance with state and federal labor laws.
- *Don't* ask the applicant his or her marital status or questions about his or her family (marital status). *Do* steer the conversation away from such topics if the applicant brings them up.
- *Don't* ask whether the applicant's religion prevents him or her from working on certain days (religion). *Do* tell the applicant the work schedule and ask if he or she is able to work at those times.
- *Don't* ask if the applicant has a disability he or she would like to disclose (disability). *Do* tell the applicant the essential functions of the job and ask if he or she is able to perform them.
- *Don't* ask the applicant if he or she has made child care arrangements (gender). *Do* tell the applicant the days and hours of work and ask if he or she can work at those times.

Q.5:4 What should an HHA do when it is ready to hire an individual?

An HHA should make an offer of employment or engagement as a subcontractor in writing. If time is of the essence, the HHA may make a verbal offer, outlining the terms of employment, and obtain a verbal commitment, following up immediately with a written offer of employment.

Q.5:5 What is the purpose and format of an offer letter?

An HHA should give any applicant it wishes to hire a written offer letter. This offer letter makes the terms of the employment clear to both the HHA and the prospective employee and allows for negotiation on certain points. The letter should contain all of the relevant points discussed during the interview. When a written offer letter is extended and accepted, the employee cannot later assert that the HHA has changed any of the terms.

In addition, the offer letter reminds the prospective employee that the employment with the HHA is on an "at-will" basis, assuming that at-will employment is viable in the particular state. Once the offer is extended and accepted in writing, the HHA should not withdraw the offer of employment, especially if the prospective employee has resigned his or her current employment. The law protects the employee who has relied upon the offer and his or her acceptance, and courts will enforce the document as if it were an employment agreement. For this reason, the HHA should ensure that the employee signs and dates the offer letter so that if problems arise, the HHA can reconcile the dates of acceptance of the new position and the resignation from the prior position. Obviously, if negative information has come to light, for example, information that the individual has a criminal conviction or a disability that prevents performance of the job, the HHA could safely rescind the offer.

If the position and its duties warrant the employee signing a noncompete agreement, the offer letter should refer to that agreement. Once the offer is accepted, the HHA should give the applicant the opportunity to look at the noncompete and have it reviewed by an attorney or other party of the applicant's choice.

An offer letter could read as follows, with each section tailored to the particular position and any specific terms agreed upon by the HHA and the prospective employee:

Date

Dear _____,

I know you will be pleased to learn that we are inviting you to join our Home Health Agency as a _____ .
Your hourly rate will be $_____, and you will also receive reimbursement for the following expenses:

_____

_____

Your hours of work will be _____

This offer of employment, as with all offers from our agency, is contingent upon a successful check of your references, a satisfactory criminal background check, and a negative test for substance abuse.

Your benefits include _____.

At the end of your 30-day probationary period, the Agency will formally evaluate your work. If both of us agree that your work is satisfactory, we will conduct a performance evaluation each year on your anniversary date. While employment is always on an at-will basis, we look forward to a long and productive association with you.

As we discussed during our interview, you will be required to sign an agreement and not to compete to protect our Agency's confidential business interests. Please review the enclosed copy.

Congratulations, and we look forward to your response by _____, with a start date of _____.

Sincerely,

Name
Title

I accept this offer of employment according to the terms within.

_____

Applicant Name   Date

_____

Manager Name   Date

EMPLOYMENT AT WILL

Q.5:6 What is employment at will?

Under the employment-at-will doctrine, if an employer and employee do not have a contract or agreement that specifies the exact term of the employment, that employment may be terminated "at will" by either party. This means that an HHA may discharge any employee at any time, with or without any plausible reason. The doctrine is not intended to give employers completely free reign, but it does allow them the flexibility to discharge employees when necessary, even if there is no obvious "good cause."

Note that the employment-at-will doctrine does not, by definition, apply to independent contractors. First, they are not employees. Second, the nature of their work lends itself to completion of specific tasks or overall projects, and when those are completed, their services may no longer be needed. Thus, there is, technically speaking, no discharge. This is one of the reasons employers often prefer to work with independent contractors.

Q.5:7 Under what conditions is the employment-at-will doctrine not valid?

The doctrine is limited in several situations. First, if an employee and employer have entered into an employment contract, the parties are bound by the terms of that contract and not by any of the concepts relating to employment at will. So if the term of the contract is one year, the employer may simply not renew and discharge the employee at that time. If the contract may be terminated for specific types of breach, such as failure to submit required reports at specific times, the employer may discharge the employee for such failure without risking a lawsuit for wrongful discharge.

In addition, an employer may not discharge an employee and claim it was done under the freedom of employment at will if that discharge was for a reason that violates public policy. For example, if the employer discharges the employee because of the employee's service on a jury or because the employee refused to perform certain illegal acts, such as falsifying records, the employee would have a claim for wrongful discharge. In addition, an HHA may not discharge an employee for reasons covered by statutes. For example, if an employee was discharged because of race or religious preference, the employee would have grounds for an action against the employer.

Q.5:8 How can an HHA ensure that the employment-at-will doctrine is not violated?

The HHA must not give any indication, either verbally or in writing, that employment is "permanent." It should ensure that its supervisory personnel do not make statements that could lead an employee to believe that employment will continue for any length of time. For example, if the agency has given the employee a satisfactory or even a glowing performance evaluation, the evaluator should never say things like "You've done so well, I'm sure you will be with us for a very long time," or "As long as you continue to do this well, I'm sure you will never be terminated." This type of statement could be used against the HHA as evidence that the HHA wished to employ the person on something other than an at-will basis.

In addition, the HHA's personnel policies must support the notion of employment at will, from the very beginning. For example, if the HHA has the employees go through an introductory or probationary period after they are first hired, it must be careful not to imply that when this period is over, the employees will be "permanent" employees. The HHA can inform a prospective employee about this in the offer letter, mentioning the probationary period and specifying that once that period is up, the HHA hopes that employment will continue but that no guarantee of continued employment is made at any time in the employment relationship.

Q.5:9 What is the status of an employee handbook?

Another place where the HHA can reinforce the at-will status of employees is in the employee handbook or manual. Many courts have supported employee claims that the employee handbook is the same as a contract for employment because it details the terms and conditions of employment and imposes duties on an employee, as a contract would. The HHA must be careful to disclaim any interpretation of the handbook as a contract and in fact to reserve to itself the right to change any of the policies, as they are primarily guides rather than binding procedures. A sample disclaimer would read thus:

> I understand and agree that the Employee Handbook does not create an employment contract. My employment is not guaranteed for any specific period and may, with or without cause, be terminated at any time without prior notice. I also understand that the Agency cannot guarantee permanent employment, nor support or enforce any promises of long-term employment made to me, either expressly or by implication, by any person associated with the Agency.

_____

Signature

_____

Date

NEGLIGENT HIRING

Q.5:10 Is an HHA liable for all of the negligent acts of its employees?

Under the doctrine of *respondeat superior*, an employer may be vicariously liable for the negligent acts of its employees. This doctrine means that even though the employee may not be immediately supervised by the employer or may not be on the employer's premises at the time a negligent act is committed, if the employee is acting on behalf of the employer or exercising the duties that the employee was hired by the employer to perform, the employer may be liable. In order for the employer to be liable, however, the act must have been committed within the scope of employment.

Q.5:11 What is negligent hiring?

Negligent hiring is a cause of action in tort by which an injured person may have a claim against an employer for negligently performing the hiring process, resulting in harm to the third party. This cause of action may extend the employer's liability to acts of the employee outside the scope of employment. Basically, the employer has a duty to use reasonable care in selecting and retaining employees. For example, an apartment complex that hires a building inspector has a duty to the tenants to verify an applicant's qualifications and character. [See *Cramer v. Housing Opportunities Commission*, 501 A.2d. 35 (1985).] In this case, the employer should have questioned why the applicant did not complete the application regarding prior discharges, should have contacted previous employers, and should have verified the information in the application. Had the employer done so, the employer might have discovered that the applicant had been convicted of violent crimes against a person and was currently under indictment for rape. Thus, when the inspector, who had easy access to the apartments, entered one of the units and assaulted and raped a tenant, the tenant brought an action against the employer. The court found in favor of the tenant, holding that information about criminal convictions is readily available and that the employer should therefore have investigated the background of the applicant before hiring him.

Q.5:12 How might negligent hiring affect an HHA?

If an HHA hires a registered nurse to provide skilled nursing services to a patient and that nurse harms the patient, either through abusive contact or perhaps theft of the patient's personal property, the patient might have a claim in tort against the HHA for negligent hiring of that nurse. The patient would have to prove that the HHA knew or should have known that there was a high probability that the nurse was going to harm the patient. For example, if the patient can prove that the HHA did no background check on the nurse and the nurse had recently had his license revoked due to abuse of a patient in another setting, the HHA could be liable for hiring that nurse without taking reasonable measures to determine his fitness for the position.

This tort grows out of a parallel theory of relief for patients who have suffered abuse of some sort by medical personnel, referred to as medical malpractice, a specific form of negligence. In one case, a medical college was sued by a patient who was abused by one of its residents. The resident had disclosed that he was a pedophiliac, and the patient charged that the college had a duty to protect the patients from this resident. The court found in favor of the patient because the actions of the resident were foreseeable and the college did not exercise reasonable care to protect the patient from the foreseeable harm. [*Almonte v. New York Medical College*, 851 F.Supp.34 (D. Conn. 1994).]

The tort of negligent hiring goes much further because it can be applied to the actions of *any* employee of an HHA, not just medical personnel. Thus, if a home health aide, a companion, a driver delivering medical equipment, or any other unlicensed individual provides care, that individual cannot be disciplined through the licensure process, and the most likely target of a lawsuit is then the HHA (because it often has the "deepest pockets"), under the theory of *respondeat superior* as well as negligent hiring.

Q.5:13 How can an HHA protect itself against negligently hiring personnel?

Home health agencies are subject to this charge even more than other types of employers because an HHA sends individuals into the home, most often with no supervision. An HHA should rigorously check its hiring process to ensure that it makes all of the appropriate investigations. The hiring person should do the following:

- Review the application carefully to reveal any gaps in employment or other inconsistencies that require further investigation.
- For licensed clinical personnel, contact the state licensing agency to verify that, indeed, the individual is licensed, ask specifically if there have been any complaints or actions against that individual's license, and ask about the outcome of any investigation.
- Contact all of the applicant's references, both personal and employment related. Also contact any other sources of information you may know about, even if the applicant has not pro-

vided their names. Obtain the applicant's consent to contact these individuals.

- Determine in advance whether the position being filled is one for which a criminal record check might be appropriate. For example, it might be appropriate for a nurse or aide who will be visiting patients in the home but not appropriate for sales representatives or clerical staff. In addition, even if the HHA does not usually perform such checks for a position, if the individual presents any suspicious information (and, for some reason, the HHA still wants to consider the applicant for employment), a criminal check might be appropriate. In any situation, inform the applicant that a criminal record check will be done and get the written consent of the applicant.
- Carefully document the results of reference checks and criminal record searches even if such checks did not reveal useful information.
- When offering employment, make the offer contingent upon a satisfactory reference and background check.

INDEPENDENT CONTRACTORS VERSUS EMPLOYEES

Q.5:14 Should an HHA hire personnel as independent contractors or as employees?

This decision should be based upon the desires and capabilities of the HHA management. For example, if the HHA wishes to maintain long-term relationships with nurses and therapists and build a stable company with well-known staff, the HHA would probably be better off hiring the staff as employees. In such a situation, all of the employment laws and practices discussed in this chapter would apply to them.

If, however, the HHA prefers not to address the myriad legal questions that arise with employees, using independent contractors may be the ideal solution. Indeed, the potential staff member may feel strongly one way or the other, and it is not uncommon for professionals to prefer independent contractor status, as they can then work for a number of different agencies.

Q.5:15 How does the IRS determine whether HHA staff are independent contractors or employees?

The IRS has developed what is known as the "common-law test," which it applies when deciding whether an individual has been working in the capacity of an independent contractor or an employee. The IRS will not take the word of the employer, as mischaracterizations cause the government to lose billions of dollars each year in unpaid employment taxes. Currently, the IRS is actively comparing the Form 1099s submitted by employers on behalf of independent contractors with those individuals' personal tax returns. If most of an individual's income derives from one source, the IRS will presume that the individual is an employee who has been misclassified as an independent contractor.

Q.5:16 What are the basic provisions of the common-law test?

Basically, the common-law test focuses on the degree of control the employer has over the performance of the work. In any working relationship, the hiring party specifies the final product to be developed, but if that party also controls the means by which the work is performed, the worker is most likely an employee. Even if the hiring party does not actually exercise control but merely has the express right to exercise control, the employment relationship may be established. If, however, the worker controls the method and specifics of performing the work, that worker is most likely an independent contractor.

The following lists contain the 20 factors developed by the IRS for the purpose of classifying independent contractors and employees:

Independent Contractors	Employees
risk of profit or loss	no risk of profit or loss
generates business independently	depends on company for work

delegates authority, hires, fires, and sets pay	has minimal powers at discretion of employer
services may be rendered by anyone	services must be rendered personally
services may be offered to the general public	services may not be offered elsewhere
services performed for several companies at one time	services performed for only (or primarily) one company at a time
services independent of company operations	work integrated into company operations
trains independently	trains with company employees, attends meetings, comunicates regularly with employees
work not controlled or supervised by company	work controlled and supervised by company
provides own work environment	company provides work area
determines own work schedule	company sets schedule
provides own tools and materials	company provides tools and materials
determines the order and method of work performed	company determines how work is performed
need not submit oral or written reports regularly	must submit regular oral or written reports
pays own expenses	company pays expenses
no fringe benefits	company provides fringe benefits
receives lump sum payments	company pays hourly wage or salary
worker cannot terminate relationship without incurring liability for product	worker can terminate relationship without incurring liability
company can discharge	company cannot discharge as long as product is satisfactory
relationship with company terminates at end of particular project	ongoing relationship with company

Q.5:17 For what other purposes may the common-law test be used?

The common-law test has proved to be a handy tool to analyze employment relationships for a number of different purposes unrelated to payroll and tax considerations. For example, the test may be used to determine whether the state workers' compensation and unemployment compensation laws apply to the individual and whether an employment relationship exists for purposes of analysis of liability for negligence and application of employment discrimination laws.

EMPLOYMENT CONTRACTS

Q.5:18 What elements are included in a contract between an HHA and its employees or subcontractors?

The contract should clearly specify whether the individual is being engaged to provide services as an employee or an independent contractor. Language to describe an employee could read as follows:

> The Company hereby agrees to employ the Employee as a home health marketing specialist, and Employee hereby accepts such employment. Employee agrees to devote full time, efforts, and skill during the term of the employment to the business of the Company and render services solely to the Company and its other employees and customers.

> The Company hereby agrees to provide the Employee with the vacation, sick, and retirement benefits according to [an attached schedule].

Language used to describe an independent contractor could read as follows (note use of the word *engagement* rather than *employment*):

The Company engages the individual's services as an independent contractor, and the individual accepts such engagement to render services as a home health marketing specialist. As an independent contractor, the means, manner, and method of the performance of the services provided by the individual under this contract shall not be under the direct supervision of the Company. The individual shall, however, be responsible to the Administrator of the Company for the quality of services provided by the individual during the term of his engagement. Further, the Company shall not be responsible for payment of any federal, state, or local income taxes, FICA, unemployment compensation or workers' compensation, vacation or sick pay, retirement benefits, or any other payments for or on behalf of the individual.

In addition, the contract should specify the following for both employees and independent subcontractors:

- special qualifications of the individual, such as licenses and continuing education credits;
- the particular duties of the individual, including the hours expected, the on-call duties, the standards of performance expected, and the nature of supervision, if any, in the performance of the duties;
- maintenance of clinical records and communication of clinical information among the various caregivers;
- the compensation due the individual under the agreement;
- maintenance of professional liability insurance;
- the term of the agreement (usually not more than one year);
- termination provisions, both "for cause" and "without cause";
- confidentiality provisions;
- an agreement, if appropriate for the particular position, not to compete with the company and not to solicit company employees or customers (see questions 5:19–5:22); and

- standard contractual provisions such as the following:
  - —a provision prohibiting the individual from assigning the contract to another individual to perform the duties;
  - —a statement identifying the governing law in case of a dispute;
  - —provisions for notice in case of termination;
  - —severability provisions, which allow the contract to remain in force even if a particular section is found to be invalid;
  - —a statement that the contract represents the total agreement of the parties and that any prior or subsequent oral discussions have no effect;
  - —indemnification for each party in the event of damages due to negligence; and
  - —if Medicare or Medicaid patients are involved, provisions allowing access to records by these programs.

COVENANTS NOT TO COMPETE

Q.5:19 What is a covenant not to compete?

A covenant not to compete, also known as a noncompetition agreement or restrictive covenant, is an agreement between an employer and its employees which in effect restricts the freedom of the individual to work for a competitor during employment and after separating from the employer. This agreement may be part of a comprehensive employment contract or a separate agreement that the employee signs even in the absence of an employment contract.

HHAs often require certain categories of employees to enter into such agreements to protect their investment in training the employees. Without a noncompete, an employee could take the experience gained at the expense of one HHA and apply it to further the interests of a competing agency. A noncompete may also specify that the employee may not solicit other employees to go to work for the new HHA, in order to protect the former HHA's investment in its employee base. Further, a noncompete should also prohibit the employee from soliciting the HHA's patients or customers as a means of protecting the HHA's patient base.

Many noncompetition agreements include a provision regarding confidentiality of HHA information above and beyond patient information. This provision covers client lists, business plans, marketing strategy, and financial information. Confidentiality provisions may be included in a noncompetition agreement because the improper disclosure of such information could adversely affect the HHA's standing in the community.

Q.5:20 What types of employees usually sign noncompetition agreements?

Generally, managerial employees and sales representatives are likely to be required to enter into such agreements. These individuals would possess significant information about the particular HHA and the industry in the area and could use such information to help competitors gain market share.

Nurses and other professionals may also be required to sign such agreements, although they should be tailored to prohibit nonsolicitation of former patients rather than rule out competition in general. In other words, a nurse may go to work for a competitor as long as he or she did not attempt to take patients to the new agency. The patients belong to the agency, loosely speaking, not to the agency employee.

In one case, an HHA charged a former employee with breach of an employment contract containing a noncompetition covenant, and charged the new employer with aiding and abetting the employee in breaching the contract. The court found that the employee did not solicit former patients, that, in fact, both she and the new agency took elaborate steps to ensure that no such solicitation could occur, but rather that the patients sought out the nurse at her new place of employment. So, too, the former coworkers of the nurse left the former employer to work for the new employer of their own free will, to continue caring for the patients that followed the nurse to the second agency. Finally, the court found that the nurse did not violate the confidentiality provisions of the employment agreement even though she had possession of activity logs because she did not show them to anyone or otherwise disclose their contents. [*Interim Health Care v. Fournier*, No. 13003, Delaware Court of Chancery, Feb. 28, 1994.]

In general, though, it may be unnecessarily duplicative to require clinical and other professional employees to enter into noncompetition agreements, as their duties are generally patient specific and patient directed and they are not likely to affirmatively compete with a former employer. In addition, they are governed by the rules of professional conduct promulgated by their professional societies and state licensing boards. Professionals can practice freely and for any clients they choose, and should a professional violate professional standards regarding, for example, confidentiality, the HHA would have recourse against that professional through his or her licensing board rather than through the courts. If, however, the bulk of the duties of, for example, a nurse are management oriented rather than clinical, the HHA should consider having the nurse sign a noncompete.

In addition, the HHA needs to keep in mind the marketing impact of this type of restriction. Even though a restriction might be legally supportable, it might be viewed negatively by prospective employees, especially if it is broadly drafted.

Q.5:21 How can an HHA ensure that a noncompetition agreement will be enforced?

The applicability of the terms of a noncompete is determined by state law, and careful drafting is required. In some states, noncompetes are prohibited by law, while in other states they are supportable if certain conditions are met. These conditions are set out in case law as exceptions to the general rule that a properly executed noncompete is legally enforceable.

Generally, though, noncompetition agreements will be construed in favor of the employee, because the employee stands to lose his or her livelihood, at least for a period of time. In addition, courts presume that even though the agreement was signed voluntarily upon obtaining employment, the employee was under a certain degree of pressure to sign the agreement. Therefore, courts will look at the following conditions when construing a noncompetition agreement:

- whether the restriction imposed upon the employee is reasonably necessary to protect the interest of the employer;
- whether the restriction imposed upon the employee is unreasonable; and
- whether the restriction imposed is against public policy.

Each case is determined on an individual basis. However, case law has provided some benchmarks for examining the restrictive effect of the agreement:

- The length of time that the restriction is effective. A restriction of six months might not be unreasonable whereas a restriction of 5 years most likely would be.
- The geographic area in which the restriction is effective. An agreement prohibiting a sales representative from selling within the area in which the HHA provides the bulk of its services would be reasonable, but prohibiting the sales representative from selling in five surrounding states is probably unreasonable. In urban areas, the extent of a reasonable area would likely be expressed in terms of number of miles from the HHA.
- The specific activity prohibited. An agreement that prohibits a sales representative from selling home health services for another agency would be reasonable, whereas an agreement that prohibits a sales representative from acting in a sales capacity in the health care field would likely be struck down by a reviewing court as being too broad.

Given these parameters, a noncompetition agreement might read as follows:

Employee acknowledges that he will be provided with confidential information of a highly sensitive and proprietary nature regarding the business of Agency. Because the disclosure of such confidential information would provide Agency's competitors with an unfair competitive advantage over Agency, Employee covenants and agrees that during the term of Employment by Agency and, except as otherwise provided herein, for a period of one (1) year after termination of Employment with Agency, within a radius of fifty (50) miles from Agency's main office or any branch office, he shall not, without prior written consent:

A. Solicit, for himself or on behalf of any person or entity, any patients or customers, or prospective patients or customers of Agency. "Patients or customers" shall mean all entities, including private individuals as well as professionals and case managers, to whom Agency has rendered its services during the period of Employee's employment by Agency. The term "prospective patients or customers" shall mean all entities who have contacted Agency, or have been contacted by Agency, within the one (1) year period prior to the date of termination of Employee's Employment.

B. Solicit, for himself or on behalf of any person or entity, any employee of Agency to work for or with Employee, or for or with any other person or entity.

C. Engage, either for himself, or for any entity, in the rendering of or consultation regarding home health services.

Q.5:22 What remedies are available to an employer if an employee violates the terms of a noncompetition agreement?

In the case of a breach of the agreement, money damages are difficult to ascertain. Thus, a noncompetition agreement will likely allow for an injunction through a court of equity. This remedy "enjoins" the former employee from continuing the new employment unless the employee provides information that the duties and scope of the employment are significantly different.

EMPLOYMENT DISCRIMINATION

Title VII of the Civil Rights Act

Q.5:23 What is Title VII and how does it affect an HHA?

Title VII of the Civil Rights Act of 1964, referred to as "Title VII," addresses the pervasive problem of employment discrimination. Title VII makes it illegal for employers to discriminate against individuals on the basis of race, religion, national origin, and sex in decisions regarding the employment relationship, including hiring, promotion, compensation, discipline, and termination decisions.

For example, if an HHA refused to hire a minority individual as a nurse because its patients expressed a preference for white nurses, the HHA would be liable for violation of Title VII's ban on racial discrimination. If, however, the HHA complied with a patient's request to have only female nurses in attendance, this would not likely be a violation of the ban on gender discrimination, due to the overriding interests of the patient's privacy.

Q.5:24 How is Title VII enforced?

Title VII is enforced by the Equal Employment Opportunity Commission (EEOC), a federal agency that enforces all of the laws that address any kind of discrimination in the workplace. In addition, states have their own antidiscrimination laws that mirror or, in some cases, are more restrictive than the federal law.

The EEOC requires employees to file a discrimination complaint within 180 days of the discriminatory event. Discriminatory events include actions on the job, such as demotion or denial of a promotion, as well as termination of employment itself. The EEOC then investigates the complaint.

If the EEOC finds that discrimination occurred, it will encourage the employer to "conciliate" the complaint, which has the effect of a settlement. The employer may offer remedies such as reinstatement and back pay or the formerly withheld promotion. If the employer refuses to conciliate, the EEOC will either file suit in court on behalf of the employee or give the employee a "letter to sue," in which case the employee has 90 days to file his or her own lawsuit. If, on the other hand, the EEOC finds that discrimination did not occur, the investigation will end and the employee still gets the letter to sue.

Sexual Harassment

Q.5:25 What is sexual harassment?

Sexual harassment is one form of discrimination on the basis of sex. As such, it is one of the types of discrimination prohibited by Title VII. In addition, many states' antidiscrimination laws address sexual harassment directly.

Title VII defines sexual harassment as

> unwelcome sexual advances, requests for sexual favors, and other verbal or physical conduct of a sexual nature . . . when:
>
> - submission to such conduct is made either explicitly or implicitly a term or condition of an individual's employment [e.g., a person's job depends on saying yes to requests for sexual favors];
> - submission to or rejection of such conduct by an individual is used as the basis for employment decision affecting such individual [e.g., a person's promotion or work assignment depends upon saying yes to a request for sexual favors]; or
> - such conduct has the purpose or effect of unreasonably interfering with an individual's work performance or creating an intimidating, hostile, or offensive working environment [e.g., a person's supervisor or coworker constantly makes jokes of a sexual nature to the person

or to coworkers when the person is around or sends suggestive notes to the person].

Q.5:26 What are the different types of sexual harassment that have been identified as illegal?

The main types of sexual harassment are known as *quid pro quo* and *hostile environment*. *Quid pro quo* literally means something given in return for something else. Thus, a supervisor who makes unwelcome sexual advances and states directly or somehow implies that the employee must either submit to the advances or be fired, lose the opportunity to perform certain tasks, or be passed over for promotion would be guilty of this type of harassment.

The hostile environment form of sexual harassment may be less obvious but is probably the most pervasive. An employee does not need to be directly approached or fired in order to be considered to have experienced sexual harassment. Courts will look at the "totality of circumstances" to determine whether the sexually suggestive conduct resulted in an environment that is hostile, abusive, or offensive. [*Meritor Savings Bank, FSB v. Vinson*, 106 S. Ct. 2399 (1986).]

In the landmark Meritor case, the Supreme Court examined whether the sexual relationship that had occurred between the plaintiff and her supervisor was voluntary. The Court said, as a basic matter, that even though the plaintiff consented to have sex with her supervisor, it was not voluntary because her job was conditioned on it. This determination, however, was not the end of the Court's inquiry; it clarified that the question to ask was whether the sexual relationship was welcome or unwelcome to the plaintiff. The major statement made in the court's opinion was that employees have the right to work in an environment free from discriminatory intimidation, ridicule, and insult. Thus, no direct advances or threats have to be made in order for sexual harassment to exist.

Q.5:27 What is the "reasonable woman" standard?

Later court cases have gone further in supporting the victims of sexual harassment. The law has generally used a "reasonable person" standard to determine, for example, whether a plaintiff should have had a certain reaction to an event, asking whether a "reasonable person," or, to some extent, an average person, would have had that reaction.

One court considered the differences between males and females in terms of what they might believe is sexually harassing behavior and established the "reasonable woman" standard. This case held that the reasonable person standard could backfire in sexual harassment cases, because if, as is asserted, sexual harassment is common, then a reasonable person could be expected to be harassed. Thus, the court said, there needs to be a special "reasonable woman" standard. Under this standard, the court recognized specifically that conduct that men may consider acceptable may upset women. Acknowledging that women are the victims of violent sexual crimes more often than men, women may have a realistic worry as to whether seemingly mild harassment may grow violent. Therefore, the different views of men and women need to be taken into account. [*Ellison v. Brady*, 924 F.2d 872 (9th Cir., 1991).]

Q.5:28 May an HHA allow employees to post sexually suggestive material in their individual work area?

Generally, no. In another 1991 case, a woman complained that pictures of nude women on the walls of the workplace were disturbing to her and other female workers. The court found that such pornographic material in the workplace conveys a message from the employer that deters women from performing well and continuing employment. [*Robinson v. Jacksonville Shipyards*, 760 F. Supp. 1486 (M.D. Fla., 1991).]

Q.5:29 What is the legal standard for measuring the extent of injury to a victim in order to determine whether sexual harassment has occurred?

The Supreme Court recently clarified that a victim need not exhibit serious psychological injury in order to win on a claim of sexual harassment. In other words, an employee need not suffer a "nervous breakdown" before harassment becomes actionable. As long as the workplace circumstances could reasonably be perceived as hostile or abusive, actual injury need not be proven. [*Harris v. Forklift Systems, Inc.*, 114 S. Ct. 367 (1993).]

The Court stressed that even though the requirement of showing psychological injury has been removed, the victim must still show that he or she perceived the environment as hostile. Thus, even if a "reasonable person" or "reasonable woman" would find the environment hostile by objective standards, the victim must still subjectively find the environment hostile although not necessarily suffering psychological injury.

Q.5:30 Can an HHA be liable for sexually harassing conduct by one employee against another or by a nonemployee against an employee?

It is clear from extensive case law, in addition to that described above, that an employer can be liable for acts of sexual harassment by one employee against another. The employer will most likely be found liable if it had actual knowledge of the actions or if, given the circumstances, it should have had knowledge. Clearly, if the victim reports the harassment to the employer and the employer takes no action, the employer is at risk.

In addition, an employer could be liable to an employee for acts of sexual harassment by a nonemployee if the HHA knew about the problem and had the power to control, or at least attempt to control, the problem. Imagine, for example, that a medical sales representative who regularly calls on the HHA makes sexually suggestive remarks to the HHA supply purchaser or receptionist, or asks her for dates or sexual favors even after being firmly told no. The supply purchaser asks that another employee meet with the sales representative, but the HHA administrator insists that there is no one else available to fill in. The supply purchaser or receptionist becomes distraught over the encounters, her performance suffers, and she is fired. She sues the HHA and will most likely win because of the poor response by the administrator.

Q.5:31 What specific actions should an HHA take to protect itself from charges of sexual harassment?

Every home health agency should develop a strongly worded policy forbidding sexual harassment in any of its forms. This policy should define the types of actions that are prohibited and the consequences for individuals who engage in sexual harassment. It should set out a particular procedure that the HHA will follow to address claims of sexual harassment, including steps for the victim to take and steps the HHA will take to discipline the harasser, beginning with a thorough investigation. The HHA must train all of its employees to recognize the problem and to avoid any actions that could be interpreted as sexually harassing behavior.

Most importantly, the HHA must follow the procedure it develops. Courts look carefully at the actions taken by an employer to combat the problem in general and in regard to specific instances in determining whether the employer attempted to deal with the situation or to look the other way. The most elaborate of procedures and the most extensive training will mean little to a court in the face of evidence showing that the employer did not acknowledge instances of sexual harassment brought to light by an employee.

Q.5:32 What steps must a victim take in order to pursue a claim for sexual harassment?

An individual who perceives herself, or possibly himself, as a victim of sexual harassment must make the problem known. The victim must prove not only that she found a coworker's advances unwelcome, or the work environment hostile, but that she actively communicated her feelings to the harasser (or asked the employer to remove offensive pictures or transfer a harassing coworker). In order to be most effective, the communication of the problem should be done in writing as well as verbally.

An HHA must create an environment in which its employees feel comfortable in bringing forth complaints within the agency so that it has an opportunity to solve the problem. If, however, the employee files a claim with the EEOC, the HHA should review its files to determine whether the employee ever informed the HHA of the problem. If not, the HHA could use the employee's inaction as a defense against the charge that it could have prevented the harassment.

Age Discrimination in Employment Act

Q.5:33 What is the Age Discrimination in Employment Act?

The Age Discrimination in Employment Act (ADEA) prohibits discrimination in employment of individuals over 40 years of age. [29 U.S.C. §623(a).] Age discrimination is the only category of discrimination not covered under Title VII. Rather, it is more closely related to the Fair Labor Standards Act in the rights and remedies it offers. Further, since passage of the Older Workers Benefit Protection Act, the ADEA expressly prohibits discrimination in employee benefits.

The law applies to companies with 20 or more employees. Under this law, any decision in which age is involved will be suspect. Mandatory retirement is prohibited except in certain circumstances.

Americans with Disabilities Act

Q.5:34 What is the Americans with Disabilities Act?

The Americans with Disabilities Act of 1990 (ADA) outlaws discrimination against a qualified individual with a disability in many facets of life. Specifically, the ADA makes it unlawful to discriminate against an individual with disabilities in state and local government services, public accommodations, transportation, telecommunications, and employment. The discussion of the ADA below focuses on the employment provisions.

Q.5:35 Which employers are covered by the ADA?

All employers with 15 or more employees are covered by the ADA. The ADA makes it unlawful for an employer to discriminate against an individual with a disability in all types of employment practices. Many of the protections afforded by the ADA were also found in the Rehabilitation Act of 1973, which applied to public employers.

The ADA, however, has extended those protections to private employers and expanded the protections as well. Although many hospital-based or government-run HHAs may have been covered under the Rehabilitation Act, the ADA clearly extends protection to employees of all HHAs.

Q.5:36 What employment practices are regulated by the ADA?

An HHA must not discriminate in any employment-related activities. This mandate affects the following practices:

- recruitment and hiring;
- training and promotion;
- firing and layoff;
- job assignments; and
- leave and benefits.

Q.5:37 Who is protected by the provisions of the ADA?

Title I of the ADA provides broad protections regarding disability. Primarily it protects "qualified individuals with a disability." Disability is defined as a physical or mental impairment that substantially limits a major life activity. In order to be "qualified" for a job, the individual must possess the skills, experience, and education to perform the essential functions of the job.

The ADA also protects individuals who have a record of having such an impairment (e.g., an individual who has recovered from cancer or had a psychiatric admission). Finally, the ADA protects those who are regarded as having an impairment (e.g., a burn victim with facial disfigurement, who may be perfectly qualified but viewed as having an impairment that may affect performance).

In addition, individuals who are associated with disabled individuals through family, business, or social relationships, whether or not disabled themselves, are protected by the act. Thus, for example, an employee who lives with a quadriplegic or a person with AIDS cannot be discriminated against because the HHA believes that the employee may have excessive absences from work due to caretaking responsibilities.

The impairment must be substantial and significantly limit or restrict a major life activity. This standard extends to hearing, seeing, speaking, breathing, performing manual tasks, walking, caring for oneself, learning, and working. Thus, an individual with epilepsy, paralysis, HIV infection, AIDS, a substantial hearing or visual impairment, mental retardation, or a specific learning disability is covered, but an individual with a minor, nonchronic condition of short duration, such as a sprain, a broken limb, or the flu, generally would not be covered.

Q.5:38 What is the "reasonable accommodation" requirement?

Reasonable accommodation is any modification or adjustment to the duties of a job or the environment in which the job is performed that will enable an individual with a disability to apply for jobs or perform essential job functions. Reasonable accommodations may include the following, depending upon the size and nature of the HHA:

- modifying equipment or the environment;
- restructuring a job or modifying work schedules;
- providing readers or interpreters; and
- allowing the employee to take leave for treatment related to the disability.

The HHA is only required to make a reasonable accommodation if the disability is known to the HHA. Thus, it is usually the employee's responsibility to disclose the disability and to request an accommodation. An employer need not make an accommodation if it would impose an undue hardship on the employer based upon objective criteria such as size and financial status of the business as compared with the cost of the accommodation.

Q.5:39 Does an HHA have to give preference to disabled individuals?

No. If it is determined that an individual is "disabled" as defined by the law, the individual must still be qualified to perform the essential functions of the job in order to be hired. The individual must possess the required employment experience, skills, licenses, or other qualifications the employer sets out for the job and must be able to perform the job with or without reasonable accommodation.

For example, assume an HHA has two qualified applicants for a nurse aide position, and one of them has a mild learning disability. Some of the essential functions of the job are lifting patients, feeding patients, refilling supplies, observing and recording patient status, and training other nurse aids. The disabled applicant may not be able to record her observations on the chart, but she is able to use a dictation device to record them and the administrative assistant can transcribe them. The HHA has met its obligation of providing a reasonable accommodation. However, this individual cannot train other nurse aides, and because this is an essential function of the job and not just a marginal function, the HHA does not have to hire her.

As another example, if the HHA refuses to hire an obese individual because the agency fears that individual might not have enough energy to make the required number of visits each day or because patients might not like being attended by an obese individual, the HHA would be in violation of the ADA. Obesity has been determined to be a protected disability under the ADA and was described by one court as a prime example of why "perceived disabilities" should be protected [*Cook v. State of Rhode Island, Department of Mental Health, Retardation and Hospitals*, 1993 EL 470697 (1st Cir.)].

Q.5:40 Under the ADA, must an HHA develop job descriptions?

No, but a written job description will be good evidence of the essential functions of the job. The job description must be prepared before an advertisement is placed or an applicant interviewed. It should contain detailed, accurate descriptions of the essential functions of the position. These essential functions, which are the main functions and not merely marginal ones, should be job related and consistent with business necessity.

Q.5:41 May an HHA require an applicant to take a medical examination?

An HHA may not ask an applicant to take a medical examination until after making a job offer. The HHA may not question the applicant about any disability but may ask the applicant whether he or she can perform specific job functions.

Once a job offer is made, the HHA can condition the offer on a satisfactory medical examination. If the examination is not satisfactory, the HHA may rescind the job offer as long as the reasons for not hiring are job related and consistent with business necessity and no reasonable accommodation could be made.

Q.5:42 May an HHA consider health and safety when deciding whether to hire an applicant or retain an employee with a disability?

Yes. If an individual poses a direct threat to him- or herself or others and that threat cannot be eliminated or reduced by a reasonable accommodation, the HHA need not hire or retain that individual. The employer must substantiate the claim of risk to health and safety through objective, medically supportable methods and not base the judgment on fear, a patronizing attitude, or stereotypes.

Q.5:43 What agency enforces the employment provisions of the ADA?

The ADA is enforced by the Equal Employment Opportunity Commission. Available remedies include hiring, reinstatement, promotion, back pay, front pay, restored benefits, reasonable accommodation, attorneys' fees, expert witness fees, and court costs.

Q.5:44 Are drug abusers and alcoholics protected by the ADA?

Current users of illegal drugs are specifically excluded from protection. An alcoholic is, however, protected under the law as long as he or she can perform the essential functions of the job. If alcohol use adversely affects job performance or conduct, the HHA may discipline, discharge, or deny employment to an alcoholic.

DRUG TESTING OF EMPLOYEES

Q.5:45 May an HHA perform drug tests on its employees?

Yes, but the HHA should perform any testing in compliance with its existing drug-testing policy.

Q.5:46 What should a drug-testing policy provide for in order to survive a legal challenge?

The policy should specify which actions are prohibited. A comprehensive policy would prohibit the following:

- Use, possession, manufacture, or distribution of illegal drugs or drug paraphernalia, unauthorized controlled substances, and alcohol.
- Reporting to work having used illegal substances or misused legal substances. Employees who test positive for drugs or alcohol should be subject to discipline, up to and including discharge. In addition, any illegal activity should be reported to law enforcement agencies. If alcohol use is allowed at an HHA-sponsored event, the HHA should reserve the right to take the necessary steps to ensure that such use is reasonable.
- Storing in a locker, desk, automobile, or other location any of the items listed above. The HHA may search these locations if it suspects the employee has stored such items.
- Refusing to consent to testing, to submit a sample for testing, or to submit to inspection when requested by HHA management.

- Switching or adulterating any sample submitted for testing.
- Conviction under any criminal drug statute for a violation occurring in the workplace.
- Failing to notify the HHA of any conviction under any criminal drug statute within five days of the conviction.
- Failing to tell the supervising nurse or administrator that the employee is using a prescribed or over-the-counter drug that may alter behavior or physical or mental ability. The supervisor or administrator must determine whether to temporarily change the employee's job assignment during the period of use.

The policy should specify the actions that the HHA will take if it suspects an employee is using drugs or alcohol. These actions, which should be communicated to the employees, may include the following:

- personal or facility searches where the presence of drugs or alcohol is indicated;
- medical evaluation, including drug testing, where behavior is erratic or judgment or performance is impaired (reasonable suspicion testing); and
- random testing, generally done off premises by a laboratory that specializes in employee drug testing.

The policy must make clear that refusal to cooperate will result in discipline, up to and including discharge.

Q.5:47 What if a supervisor hears from a third party that an employee may be abusing drugs or alcohol?

The supervisor should personally observe the behavior. Once it has been observed, the HHA can decide the proper course of action. If the employee has substances in his or her possession, the HHA may take appropriate disciplinary action as outlined in the policy, up to and including discharge. If, however, the supervisor observes *use* of substances and not mere possession, the HHA should send the employee for a drug test.

Q.5:48 What behaviors should alert supervisors that a drug test may be necessary?

Several types of behaviors and incidents may justify directing an employee to take a test for substance abuse. A supervisor should not order a test unless he or she has *directly* observed the behavior, either independently or after being informed that the behavior may have occurred. The information may come from a patient, customer, or coworker. Testing would be justified by any of the following:

- use of alcohol or drugs;
- possession of alcohol or drug paraphernalia;
- signs and symptoms of alcohol or drug use, such as slurred speech and odor of alcohol on breath;
- an accident or incident in which misuse of drugs or use of illegal substances is indicated; and
- deteriorating job performance or erratic on-the-job behavior.

Q.5:49 What are acceptable procedures for testing employees suspected of substance abuse?

Once a supervisory nurse or administrator has observed and verified that one of the above behaviors or incidents has occurred, he or she should follow specific steps outlined in a policy. If at any point in the procedure the employee does not cooperate, the employee is in violation of agency policy and the supervisor must implement the standard disciplinary procedure.

The supervisor should prepare a confidential written memorandum for approval by the administrator, describing the circumstances justifying the referral for the alcohol or drug test.

The supervisor should inform the employee of the reason for testing, focusing directly on the deteriorating job performance or other problem behavior; review the agency's alcohol and drug abuse policy and its testing procedures; and obtain the employee's consent to be tested.

The supervisor should immediately schedule an appointment with the laboratory for the employee to be tested, telling the employee the name and address of the laboratory. If the employee is combative or the supervisor feels that the employee may become combative, the supervisor should request police support.

The supervisor should explain that the employee will be placed on leave without pay pending investigation following the results of the test. If the test results are negative, the employee will be paid for the time absent from work.

Once the employee has been fully informed regarding the testing, the supervisor should call a taxicab to take the employee to the laboratory at the agency's expense. The supervisor should escort the employee to the taxicab and inform the employee that he or she must present appropriate photo identification (photo ID, driver's license, etc.) at the laboratory. The HHA should also pay for a taxicab to take the employee home after the test. The employee should be instructed not to report to work until the supervisor contacts him or her.

The procedures for obtaining and testing the sample at the laboratory should be performed in accordance with all federal and state laws governing laboratories.

Once test results have been received, the supervisor should consult with the administrator to determine the appropriate disciplinary action. If the test results are negative, those individuals should decide whether appropriate disciplinary action is necessary to resolve problems that are causing deteriorating job performance or erratic on-the-job behavior. If the investigation does not result in the employee's discharge, he or she will be reinstated with full pay and benefits.

The HHA must be careful to keep all information regarding testing in strictest confidence. All records relating to the drug and alcohol tests should be locked in a file in the office of the administrator, who will be the only individual with access to the file. Only the supervisor and the administrator are deemed to have a "need to know" an employee's test results. If the employee is discharged because of a confirmed positive result on a substance abuse test, other employees should not be told the reason for the discharge. If an explanation is necessary, it should be restricted to the statement that the employee was discharged for medical reasons.

Q.5:50 What possible legal challenges may an HHA face if it chooses to test its employees?

The most commonly discussed causes of action regarding drug testing are constitutional challenges, usually the Fourth Amendment search and seizure argument. A constitutional argument, however, is possible only when the testing is done on public-sector employees, as it applies only to state action. Private-sector testing will not have the state action component necessary to invoke constitutional protection.

Employees in the private sector are enormously creative, however, and can pursue any number of theories in their quest to elude employment-related consequences of abusing drugs or alcohol. For example, employees may allege one of the following:

- defamation, if the HHA informs third parties incorrectly that a drug test was done when it was not or that a result was positive when it was not and the employee cannot find work due to the injury to his or her reputation;
- infliction of emotional distress, if the HHA or the laboratory treated the employee improperly during the drug-testing process; and
- invasion of privacy, if the HHA disclosed the test results improperly.

THE FAMILY AND MEDICAL LEAVE ACT

Q.5:51 How does the Family and Medical Leave Act apply to an HHA?

The Family and Medical Leave Act of 1993 (FMLA) requires employers of 50 or more employees to grant up to 12 weeks of unpaid leave per year, or paid leave if it has been earned, to employees who need to care for themselves or for family members who have serious illnesses. An HHA is covered by the law if there were 50 or more employees employed for each working day during 20 or more calendar workweeks in the current or preceding year. [See 29 U.S.C. §§2601 *et seq.*; 58 *Federal Register* 31813 *et seq.*, Interim Regulations (June 4, 1993).]

If an HHA is a division or branch of a larger entity, it may, even if it itself does not have 50 employees, be covered by the act if it meets the definition of an "integrated employer." The FMLA lists specific factors to consider in determining whether two entities should be viewed as one integrated employer:

- common management;
- interrelation between operations;
- centralized control of labor relations; and
- degree of common ownership and financial control.

A determination of whether these factors are present is not achieved through the application of any single criterion; rather the entire relationship is reviewed in its totality. In addition, even if an HHA is not covered by the FMLA, many states have enacted family leave laws, so agencies should check their state's law.

Q.5:52 Who is entitled to take FMLA leave?

An "eligible" employee is one who has been employed by the employer for at least 12 months prior to the leave request and who has at least 1,250 hours of service with that employer during the prior 12 months. The act does not apply to independent contractors, although it would apply to employees working under a negotiated employment agreement. Males as well as females are eligible to take leave.

Q.5:53 If a branch office has fewer than 50 employees, is that branch office covered?

If the HHA has branches with less than 50 employees, these work sites are not covered, although the main office or other branches with more than 50 employees are still covered. If, however, the HHA has a total of 50 or more employees within 75 miles of a smaller work site, then the HHA must provide leave to the employees of the smaller site. Presumably, the other site or sites would be in a position to send employees to the smaller site to cover the duties of the employee on leave. For employees who have no fixed work site, their work site is considered to be the single site of employment to which they are assigned as their home base, from which their work is assigned, or to which they report.

For purposes of counting employees to meet the 50-employee threshold, all employees who are on the payroll for the week in which the count is done must be counted. This includes part-time employees as well as those on leaves of absence.

Q.5:54 Must an HHA hold an employee's position open during FMLA leave?

The intent behind the FMLA is to help employees balance family needs and their need for employment and related benefits. To this end, an HHA must restore a returning employee to the same or an equivalent position with equivalent pay, benefits, and other terms and conditions of employment. If during the leave the HHA had to fill the position, the employee must be placed in another position at the same rate of pay he or she would have earned had he or she remained at work, even if that position does not pay as much as the employee was earning.

If the employee is among the highest paid 10 percent of employees, or a "key" employee, the HHA may deny restoration of the position as long as it notifies the employee of its intent to deny restoration as soon as that decision is made.

Q.5:55 Must an HHA continue an employee's benefits?

An HHA must continue an employee's health insurance under the same conditions as if the employee were working. In this situation, the employee will still be required to pay his or her share of the premium if the plan provides for such copayments. If prior to the leave request the employer was paying the employee's premium in full, the employer may not then require the employee to contribute.

Should the employee decide not to return to work for reasons other than a continuation of the medical problem that necessitated the leave, or if the employee returns to work for less than 30 days, the HHA may recover any premiums it paid on behalf of the employee. If the employee took paid leave for some part of the leave period, the HHA may not recover the premiums that were paid during the period of paid leave.

In addition, the HHA must maintain the other benefits accrued before the leave started, including leave, life or disability insurance, educational benefits, and pensions.

Q.5:56 For what types of conditions and for which family members may an employee take leave?

An employee may take leave for care of the employee's new child (birth, adoption, or placement for foster care). Leave for this purpose must be taken within 12 months of the birth or placement of the child. Both male and female employees may take leave for this reason. In addition, an expectant mother may take leave before the birth of the child for prenatal care or if her condition makes her unable to work. Adoptive or foster parents may also take leave before the actual placement of the child if absence from work is required for the placement or adoption to proceed.

An employee may also take leave to act as a caregiver if the employee's spouse, or a child or parent develops a serious health condition. The range of family members covered by this provision includes biological and step children under 18, any individual who functioned as a parent to the employee when the employee was a child, and any child for whom the employee functions as a parent. It does not include parents-in-law. It also includes children over the age of 18 who are incapable of self-care because of a mental or physical disability. Both male and female employees may take leave for this reason.

Finally, an employee may take leave if he or she has a serious health condition that prevents performance of the functions of his or her position. This standard is higher than that for care of family members, and thus while the employee may take leave to care for an ill parent even if the parent is not completely debilitated, that same employee would have to be completely unable to perform his or her job in order to take leave for his or her own serious health condition. For example, an employee receiving chemotherapy may be physically and mentally capable of performing the job duties and may continue to work while receiving treatment. The time taken to receive treatments or needed for follow-up visits will be covered, but the employee will be expected to report to work at other times.

Q.5:57 What is meant by the term "serious health condition"?

A serious health condition involves inpatient care and a period of condition-related incapacity or treatment. The incapacity or treatment must require an absence of more than three days from work, school, or other daily activities, and continuing or recurring treatment (two or more visits) by a health care provider. Short-term conditions are not included unless they develop into serious health conditions as a result of complications.

Examples of serious health conditions include pregnancy, cancer, cardiovascular conditions, allergies, stress and other psychological conditions, substance abuse, back conditions requiring extensive therapy or surgical procedures, and acute illnesses such as appendicitis or gallstones. Employees need not be given FMLA leave for voluntary or cosmetic treatment, routine preventive physical examinations, or absences due to substance abuse without treatment.

Q.5:58 Who qualifies as a health care provider?

Health care providers include doctors of medicine or osteopathy, podiatrists, dentists, clinical psychologists, optometrists, chiropractors, nurse practitioners, nurse midwives, and Christian Science practitioners.

Q.5:59 How may FMLA leave be taken?

An employee may take FMLA leave in any type of arrangement that is practicable for the employee and the HHA. Leave may be taken all at once or in segments of weeks or days or even hours (segmented leave is referred to as intermittent or reduced schedule leave). For example, if chemotherapy is required three times per week for three hours at a time, the employee would use nine hours per week of the total allotment of 12 weeks.

Q.5:60 What notice must an employee give to take FMLA leave?

The employee must give the HHA at least 30 days' notice if the need for leave is foreseeable, as in the case of a birth. If the need for leave is not foreseeable, the employee must give notice as soon as practicable. Where possible, the employee must make a reasonable effort not to unduly disrupt the employer's operations.

Q.5:61 What notice must an HHA give of the basic provision of the FMLA?

The HHA must post a notice prepared or approved by the Department of Labor that describes the basic provisions of the FMLA. The notice need not be a separate notice but can be provided with other notices required by law.

Q.5:62 May an HHA require medical certification to support the request for leave?

The HHA may not require medical certification for the birth or placement of a child; the entitlement to 12 weeks is absolute for this event. The HHA may require certification if the leave is for a serious health condition (either of a family member or of the employee). If the HHA has reason to doubt the validity of the certification, it may require, at its own expense, a second opinion from a provider not regularly employed by the HHA. If the first and second opinions differ, the HHA may require, again at its own expense, the opinion of a third health care provider selected and approved by both the HHA and employee. This third opinion is final and binding on both the HHA and the employee.

Q.5:63 What remedies are available to its employees if an HHA violates the law?

The secretary of labor has investigative authority provided under the Fair Labor Standards Act. The secretary will investigate and attempt to resolve complaints of violations.

An employee can sue the HHA if the HHA interferes with the employee's exercise of rights under the FMLA. The employee may seek damages in the amount of any wages, salary, employment benefits, or other compensation denied or lost because of a violation, plus interest. In addition, the employee may be awarded liquidated damages equal to the sum of the amount awarded and interest. The employee may also seek relief in a court of equity, which means that instead of monetary damages, the employee may receive employment, reinstatement, and promotion, where applicable. Attorneys' fees are also available.

Congress was serious when it enacted the FMLA, as evidenced by the additional remedies available to employees. An employee may

bring suit for damages or equitable relief in federal or state court, for and on behalf of themselves or for themselves and other employees similarly situated. Even more interestingly, the secretary of labor may sue the employer, with any damages held in an account and paid directly to each employee affected. The secretary may also seek injunctive relief, obtaining pay, benefits, interest, employment, reinstatement, and promotion, where applicable.

EMPLOYEE COMPENSATION

Q.5:64 What is the Fair Labor Standards Act and how does it affect an HHA?

A home health agency, like any business, must comply with the provisions of the Fair Labor Standards Act (FLSA). [29 U.S.C. §§201–219 (1988).] The FLSA is the leading federal law addressing compensation, specifically wages and overtime compensation. Virtually every home health agency will find itself subject to the FLSA's requirements. Either the HHA itself as an entity will be covered or its employees will be protected by the provisions of the FLSA.

The basic concepts embodied in the provisions of the FLSA are very simple:

- Employees must be paid a minimum wage per hour worked.
- Employees must be paid overtime wages at the rate of 1.5 times their regular hourly rate for any hours worked in excess of 40 hours in a workweek.

Q.5:65 How are the calculations made under the FLSA?

The HHA must determine the employee's workweek, the employee's regular rate of pay, and the actual hours worked in order to calculate the amount of payment due the employee.

- *Workweek.* A workweek is basically seven consecutive 24-hour periods. The workweek can begin on any day of the week and will end seven days later. It can mirror the HHA's payroll

period or can be completely independent of the payroll or any other measure of time. The workweek may vary for different employees as long as it remains constant for each employee (this is for purposes of calculating payment for hours worked).

- *Regular rate of pay.* The regular rate of pay may vary from the hourly wage paid to the employee. It is, rather, the hourly rate the employee is actually paid for hours worked. The amount can change as the number of hours worked changes.
- *Hours worked.* The calculation of wages and overtime is based upon hours actually worked, and thus this calculation is central to the application of the FLSA. The FLSA defines "hours worked" as the time for which an employee is entitled to compensation. [29 C.F.R. §§778.223, 785.11-13.] This includes:
  —all time during which the employee is required to be on duty or on the employer's premises or at a particular workplace;
  —all time during which the employee is "suffered or permitted" to work whether or not he or she is required to do so;
  —work not requested but suffered or permitted, even if performed away from the HHA's premises or worksite or at the employee's home; and
  —idle time or time spent on activities incidental to the work ordered by the HHA or on unproductive work.

Q.5:66 How can an HHA avoid paying an employee overtime wages?

In order for an HHA to avoid paying overtime wages to an employee, the HHA must be able to prove that the employee is "exempt" from overtime under the FLSA. The most common exemption is that for executive, administrative, and professional employees. Whether a particular employee meets the test for this exemption depends upon the nature of the employee's duties, the supervisory responsibilities, and the compensation received for services performed. Moreover, classification of the employee as exempt without any supporting evidence, such as a job description and actual duties indicating a "white-collar" type of job, will not

preserve the exemption for the HHA, and the agency may end up paying overtime and back salary as well as penalties for misclassification.

Registered nurses and licensed therapists who perform their professional duties would likely be exempt from overtime, whereas practical nurses, home health aides, and therapy assistants would not be exempt. The RNs and therapists are most often paid on a salary basis, and the assistants are paid on an hourly basis.

Q.5:67 What is the significance of paying employees a salary rather than on an hourly basis?

Generally, an employee who is paid on an hourly basis will not qualify as an exempt employee, and the HHA must pay overtime for any hours worked in excess of 40 hours in a workweek. In order to avoid liability for overtime, the HHA must pay the employee on a salary basis. While virtually all exempt employees are paid on a salary basis, however, not all employees paid on a salary basis are exempt.

For example, a supervisor may be paid on a salary basis as a reward for a job well done and an indication that further promotion is likely, but that supervisor may not be exempt from overtime if his or her duties do not conform to the type described in the FLSA for exempt employees. Conversely, some licensed therapists may prefer to be paid on an hourly basis so that they can, in fact, receive overtime pay, and this is legally permissible, although perhaps not sound from a business point of view. As long as the HHA does not pay them on an hourly basis and then still try to justify their exempt status, there should be no adverse consequences.

The final type of payment for exempt employees is the "fee basis" of payment. Under this method, the employee is paid an agreed sum for a single unique job. Payment is made regardless of the time it takes for the task to be completed.

Q.5:68 What is the status of the per-visit method of payment under the FLSA?

Many HHAs pay for some or all their nursing services on a per-visit basis. Under this method, the HHA combines all aspects of each visit in the compensation, including the travel to and from the patient's home, the actual services provided to the patient, the paperwork, and the conferences with other caregivers. Whether a per-visit payment is a type of fee, qualifying the individual for the exemption from overtime, is difficult to ascertain.

Under the FLSA, payment on a fee basis qualifies employees for the administrative or professional exemption from overtime. The regulations specify that payments made for a task that is "unique" would qualify as fee-basis payments, while payments based on the number of hours or days worked, as opposed to the completion of a task, are not fee-basis payments. If the home health agency paid the nurse additional wages for tasks outside the scope of the visit, it would appear that the nurse was nonexempt and would thus be due overtime if the hours worked exceeded 40. Conversely, agencies should not attempt to pay an employee who is nonexempt (i.e., usually paid hourly) on a per-visit basis with the goal of having that employee be exempt and therefore avoiding overtime.

Q.5:69 How must HHAs pay employees who provide companionship services?

Many HHAs offer companionship services in addition to skilled nursing and therapy services, and the employees who provide such services are exempt from the minimum wage and overtime require-ments of the FLSA. [29 C.F.R. §552.2.] The regulations interpreting the FLSA refer to these services as "companionship services for the aged or infirm," and define them as

> those services which provide fellowship, care and protec-tion for a person who, because of advanced age or physical or mental infirmity, cannot care for his or her own needs. Such services may include household work related to the care of the aged or infirm person such as meal preparation, bed making, washing of clothes, and other similar services. They may also include the performance of general house-hold work. *Provided, however,* that such work is incidental,

i.e., does not exceed 20 percent of the total weekly hours worked. . . [29 C.F.R. §552.6.]

In order for the HHA to be exempt from the FLSA requirements, all of the above criteria must be met. First, the services must be merely companionship services, not skilled services, and they must be provided to the patient and not the caregivers. [29 C.F.R. §552.106.] In addition, the patient must be unable to care for him- or herself.

The activities that can be construed as "general household work" may not account for more than 20 percent of the total hours worked. These activities include household chores not directly related to the personal care of the patient, such as washing the floors, vacuuming, dusting, and cleaning the refrigerator or oven. Even if the employee works in excess of 40 hours per week, if this type of work does not exceed 20 percent of the total hours worked, the HHA does not need to observe the minimum wage and overtime provisions.

Further, the regulation specifically addresses the question of "employees who are engaged by an employer or agency other than the family or household using their services," such as an HHA, and clarifies that such employees are exempt from the FLSA's requirements. [29 C.F.R. §552.109.]

Q.5:70 What if companionship services are provided by skilled personnel?

The regulation specifically provides that the scope of the meaning of "companionship services" "does not include services relating to the care and protection of the aged or infirm which require and are performed by trained personnel, such as a registered or practical nurse." Thus, skilled services are not included in the definition of companionship. Even though, for example, home health aides may provide companionship services, and those aides are "trained," in that they complete training courses required by the Medicare program or state programs, they are not considered "trained" as this term is used in the companionship services exemption. Therefore, home health aides delivering services that fit the definition of companionship services still qualify for the exemption from the FLSA requirements.

SAFETY

Q.5:71 What is OSHA?

The Occupational Safety and Health Act [29 U.S.C. §§651 *et seq.*] governs on-the-job safety. It generally requires employers to provide a workplace that is free from recognized hazards that cause or are likely to cause death or serious injury and to meet various standards developed as a means to provide a safe workplace. OSHA requires employers to undertake extensive training in safety measures appropriate to the particular workplace.

Q.5:72 Are there any special rules that address the health care industry?

OSHA has developed standards that apply specifically to employees of health care facilities, who are, by the nature of their contact with patients, at risk for exposure to communicable diseases. [29 C.F.R. Part 1910.1030 Subpart Z.] These standards, known as the Bloodborne Pathogen Standards, address the occupational exposure to hepatitis B virus (HBV) and human immunodeficiency virus (HIV) as well as other bloodborne diseases such as syphilis, malaria, babesiosis, brucellosis, leptospirosis, arboviral infections, relapsing fever, Creutzfeldt-Jakob disease, human T-cell lymphotrophic virus Type 1, and viral hemorrhagic fever. Their status vis-à-vis home health agencies is unclear at this point, although it is likely that HHAs will be subject to these rules; even if they are not, the requirements are worthwhile for an HHA to be aware of.

The standards focus on identifying health care workers with substantial risk of exposure and providing them the appropriate training, personal protective equipment, and vaccination. This is a marked departure from traditional infection control rules, which focus on the prevention and management of infection in the patient population. Given the risk criteria, HHA administrative staff, whose level of patient contact, and therefore risk, is no greater than that of the general population, may not be subject to the OSHA requirements.

Q.5:73 What specific actions are required under the regulations?

Each health care facility must develop a plan to assess and address its particular risks and then implement the plan throughout the facility. The plan must address the following:

- identification of jobs and job tasks that are likely to result in exposure;
- development of procedures to ensure compliance with rules regarding universal precautions (discussed below);
- a program for hepatitis B vaccination;
- use of signs, labels, and informational publications to identify hazards; and
- development of procedures for analyzing incidents of exposure.

The core of the standards is the set of procedures referred to as "universal precautions." These precautions should be taken by all employees who have contact with patients, patients' blood, or other bodily fluids. Thus, nurses, physicians, home health aides, and therapists who attend patients in the home setting should adhere to the following universal precautions:

- Assume that blood and all other bodily fluids from all patients are infectious.
- Wash hands before and after contact with each patient.
- Wear gloves, a gown, and a mask when contact with blood, body fluid, tissues, mucous membranes, or surfaces contaminated by any of these fluids is possible or when there is a break in your skin.
- Handle sharp objects with care. Do not reuse needles, and observe safety procedures for inserting new needles. Discard

sharps immediately after use into an impervious container designed specifically for sharps.

- Use mouthpieces, resuscitation bags, and other resuscitation devices when performing resuscitation.
- Clean up all spills and isolate the area until the cleanup is complete.
- Post signs reminding employees to use universal precautions in appropriate areas.
- Report all needle sticks, spills, sprays of fluids, and contamination of open wounds.

6

Medicare Reimbursement

As this book goes to press, there is no aspect of Medicare reimbursement for home health care services that is not undergoing serious scrutiny. Utilization of the home health and related services by Medicare beneficiaries has increased dramatically in response to cost-containment measures instituted by hospitals and the resulting shorter lengths of stay. From the conditions of participation, to the reasonable-cost reimbursement methodology, to the restructuring of the home health benefit (including possible requirement of a copayment by beneficiaries), reimbursement for home health care will see many changes in the future. Any changes that occur, however, will be based upon the current principles of coverage and reimbursement, and agencies need to be familiar with these basic principles. As always, agencies need to be vigilant to ensure that they in no way operate in a manner that could be considered as fraudulent or abusive.

COVERAGE OF HOME HEALTH SERVICES

Q.6:1 What types of home health services are covered under Medicare?

The term "home health services" embraces the following items and services:

- part-time or intermittent nursing care provided by or under the supervision of a registered professional nurse;
- physical, occupational, or speech therapy;

- medical social services provided under the direction of a physician;
- part-time or intermittent services of a home health aide;
- medical supplies (including catheters, catheter supplies, ostomy bags, and supplies related to ostomy care but excluding drugs and biologicals) and the use of durable medical equipment; and
- in the case of an HHA affiliated with or under common control of a hospital, medical services provided by an intern or a resident-in-training of that hospital under an approved teaching program. [42 U.S.C. §1395x(m); 42 C.F.R. §409.40.]

Q.6:2 Why are skilled nursing and therapy services required as part of the home health benefit?

Restricting the home health benefit to individuals who require some skilled nursing services or therapy services ensures that the benefit is not merely a long-term custodial benefit. In this way, the utilization of home health services remains consonant with the purpose of the Medicare program, which is to provide health care, not merely custodial care, to the aged.

Q.6:3 What types of services are specifically excluded from coverage?

The following services are explicitly excluded from coverage:

- services or items that would not be paid for in the inpatient hospital setting, including private duty nursing and items of comfort not necessary for treatment, such as television;
- services of housekeepers;
- food service arrangements, such as Meals-on-Wheels programs; and
- transportation required to take homebound individuals to a hospital, SNF, rehabilitation center, or other place to receive services that cannot be provided in the home. [42 C.F.R. §409.40.]

THE PROVIDER AGREEMENT

Q.6:4 What must an HHA do to become a provider of services under Medicare?

In order to participate in Medicare, the HHA must meet the definition of "home health agency" as set out in the Social Security Act. [42 U.S.C. §1395x(o).]

The term "home health agency" means a public agency or private organization, or a subdivision of such an agency or organization, which

1. is primarily engaged in providing skilled nursing services and other therapeutic services;
2. has policies established by a group of professional personnel (associated with the agency or organization), including one or more physicians and one or more registered professional nurses, to govern the services (referred to in paragraph (1)), which it provides, and provides for supervision of such services by a physician or a registered professional nurse;
3. maintains clinical records on all patients;
4. in the case of an agency or organization in any State in which State or applicable local law provides for the licensing of agencies or organizations of this nature, (A) is licensed pursuant to such law, or (B) is approved, by the agency of such State or locality responsible for licensing agencies or organizations of this nature, as meeting the standards established for such licensing;
5. has in effect an overall plan and budget prepared under the direction of the governing body of the institution, including an annual operating budget, a three-year capital expenditures plan, and annual review and updating [see 42 U.S.C. §1395x(z)];

6.   meets the conditions of participation as the Secretary may find necessary in the interest of the health and safety of individuals who are furnished services by such agency or organization;

7.   meets such additional requirements (including conditions relating to bonding or establishment of escrow accounts, as the Secretary finds necessary for the financial security of the program) as the Secretary finds necessary for the effective and efficient operation of the program.

In addition to these requirements, the HHA must be in compliance with Title VII of the Civil Rights Act of 1964 and must sign a participation agreement with the secretary. [Soc. Sec. Act §1861.]

Q.6:5 What is a provider agreement?

Also known as a participation agreement, it is an agreement between HCFA and a health care provider to provide services to Medicare beneficiaries and to comply with the requirements of Section 1866 of the Social Security Act. [42 C.F.R. §489.3.] When an HHA applies for participation, HCFA will determine whether the conditions of participation have been met, the civil rights requirements are met, and the HHA appropriately offers information regarding advance directives.

If HCFA accepts the HHA as a participant, it will send the HHA written notice of that determination and two copies of the provider agreement. An official of the HHA must sign both copies and return them to HCFA, which will return one copy to the HHA, indicating the dates on which it was signed by the HHA and accepted by HCFA as well as the effective date of the agreement.

The effective date of the agreement is the date the survey is completed successfully or the date on which the HHA submits a correction plan acceptable to HCFA and/or an approvable waiver request, whichever is earlier. [42 C.F.R. §489.11–13.]

Q.6:6 How does Medicare determine if it should grant an application for participation?

Medicare will only pay for services that meet conditions of coverage and are delivered by providers that meet the conditions of participation. The secretary of health and human services makes this determination, but as it would be impossible for the secretary to personally review all of the applications and inspect the providers' facilities and operations, the secretary is required to enter into an agreement with any state willing and able under which the state will certify whether the provider meets Medicare standards. In practice, most states willingly enter into such agreements, usually between the state health department and the secretary.

In order to implement this requirement, an HHA provider agreement must include a provision that the HHA may be subject to a standard survey by a state or local agency without any notice. That agency must conduct a survey at least once every 15 months, and more often if there are complaints about the quality of services or if there has been a change of ownership. If the results of the survey show that the HHA provided substandard care, the agency will perform an extended survey in which the agency and the HHA identify and review the causes of the problem.

Q.6:7 What is the status of the state certification survey?

Certification by the state survey agency that a provider meets Medicare conditions of coverage or participation represents only a recommendation to HCFA. Such certification does not guarantee that HCFA will decide that the provider is eligible to participate in or be covered under the Medicare program. HCFA makes its own independent determination and sends a notice of that determination to the provider. [42 C.F.R. §488.12.]

Any HHA accredited by the Community Health Accreditation Program (CHAP), however, may be "deemed" Medicare-certified. That is, the HHA will automatically be Medicare-certified without a second survey. CHAP notifies HCFA if the HHA wishes to take advantage of its deemed status.

Q.6:8 On what grounds may HCFA deny a provider agreement?

HCFA may decline to accept an HHA's provider agreement on the following grounds:

- The principals of the HHA have been convicted of fraud;
- The HHA has failed to disclose ownership and control interests;
- The HHA cannot give satisfactory assurance of compliance with the requirements of Title XVIII of the act; or
- The HHA is not in compliance with civil rights requirements. [42 C.F.R. §489.12.]

In addition, if HCFA determines that an HHA is no longer in compliance with the conditions of participation or coverage based upon the state survey and terminates the provider agreement, the provider may appeal the determination.

Q.6:9 How does an HHA appeal an initial denial for participation in Medicare?

If HCFA determines that an HHA is not in compliance with the conditions of participation, and, therefore, cannot participate in Medicare, the HHA may file a written request for reconsideration with HCFA or the state survey agency within 60 days from the date it received the notice of the adverse determination. The request for reconsideration must state the issues or the findings of fact with which the HHA disagrees and the reasons for disagreement. HCFA will review written evidence regarding the initial determination and make a reconsidered determination, which is binding unless further revised by HCFA or reversed or modified by a hearing decision. [42 C.F.R. §489.22.]

Q.6:10 How does an HHA appeal an initial determination to terminate its provider agreement?

A current Medicare provider that is terminated from the program for noncompliance need not go through the reconsideration process but may proceed directly to a hearing with an administrative law judge.

Q.6:11 What other types of initial determinations are made regarding program participation?

The Office of Inspector General (OIG) makes initial determinations with respect to the termination of a provider agreement due to suspension, exclusion, or denial of reimbursement because of fraud or abuse or conviction of crimes related to participation in the program. HHAs whose provider agreements are terminated for these reasons do not have the right to reconsideration of these determinations. [42 C.F.R. §489.22.]

Q.6:12 What happens to its provider agreement if an HHA is sold or new investors become involved after the agreement is signed?

If the HHA is contemplating or negotiating a change of ownership, the HHA must notify HCFA. At the occurrence of the change in ownership, the existing provider agreement will automatically be assigned to the new owner in order to minimize any disruption to the beneficiaries. The new owners will be subject to any conditions upon the agreement. [42 C.F.R. §484.19.]

A recent case has cast doubt upon the principle of automatic assignment of the provider number to a new owner. In *U.S. v. Vernon Home Health Care, Inc.* (93-4621 [5th Cir. June 1994]), the court ruled that the buyer was liable for the seller's Medicare overpayment because the buyer had accepted automatic assignment of the HHA's Medicare provider number. The buyer did so to minimize disruption to the agency's patients that might have occurred had the buyer applied for a new provider number. The agreement to sell the HHA in *Vernon* went so far as to specify that the buyer was not assuming any liabilities. The Supreme Court refused to hear the case, but other appeals courts are likely to challenge HCFA if it continues to recoup overpayments from other buyers. It is also possible that HCFA will amend its regulations regarding change of ownership to allow the buyer and seller to agree that the seller should remain responsible for any overpayments. Thus, pending resolution of this issue, it may be advisable for a buyer to get its own provider number.

Q.6:13 What are the essential provisions of a provider agreement?

When entering into a provider agreement, the HHA agrees to the following terms:

1. The HHA agrees to limit its charges to beneficiaries and to other individuals on their behalf to the costs of noncovered services, the deductible, coinsurance, and copayment amounts. [42 C.F.R. §489.20.] The HHA may not charge a beneficiary for services for which the provider is entitled to payment under Medicare or for services for which the beneficiary would have been entitled to have payment made had the HHA had the correct documentation regarding physician certification and amounts due on behalf of the individual. [42 C.F.R. §489.21.]

2. The HHA agrees to make adequate provision for the return or other disposition of any amounts incorrectly collected from a beneficiary or any person on his or her behalf. "Incorrectly collected" means that the individual is found to be retroactively entitled to benefits even though the individual has already paid for the services. Payment to the beneficiary must be made within 60 days, and any amounts not properly returned may be offset against amounts otherwise due the provider. [42 C.F.R. §489.41.]

3. The HHA agrees to notify HCFA if it hires any individual who, at any time during the preceding year, was employed

in a managerial, accounting, auditing, or similar capacity by an intermediary that services the HHA. This requirement applies to all branches of the HHA as well as to the home office.

4. The HHA agrees to furnish supplies related to ostomy care to any individual who requires them as part of its furnishing of home health services. [42 C.F.R. §489.20.]

5. The HHA agrees to develop written policies and procedures regarding advance directives.

Q.6:14 How may a provider agreement be terminated?

The provider agreement may be terminated by either the provider, HCFA, or the OIG.

Q.6:15 What if the provider decides to terminate the provider agreement?

If the provider decides to terminate the agreement, it must give notice to HCFA. The effective date must be the first day of a month, and generally it will be 6 months after the notice is given. However, if a provider ceases to provide services to the community, the date on which services ceased is the effective date of termination of the agreement. The provider must give public notice at least 15 days before the effective date of termination by publication in the newspaper. The notice must specify that payment is available for up to 30 days after the effective date of termination for home health services furnished under a plan established before the effective date of termination. [42 C.F.R. §489.52.]

Q.6:16 Under what circumstances may HCFA terminate the provider agreement?

HCFA may terminate the provider agreement if it determines any of the following regarding the HHA:

- The HHA is not complying with the provisions of Title XVIII and the regulations or with the provisions of the provider agreement.
- The HHA no longer meets the conditions of participation.
- The HHA restricts who it will accept for treatment and either does not exempt Medicare beneficiaries from that restriction or does not apply it to Medicare beneficiaries the same as to all other persons seeking treatment.
- The HHA refuses to furnish information to HCFA or permit HCFA to examine its records in order for HCFA to determine payment amounts.
- The HHA failed to disclose information on ownership or regarding convicted individuals.
- The HHA failed to comply with civil rights requirements. [42 C.F.R. §489.53.]

Q.6:17 Under what circumstances may the Office of Inspector General terminate the provider agreement?

The OIG may terminate the provider agreement (i.e., exclude the provider from program participation) if the OIG finds that the HHA has engaged in fraud or abuse. The OIG must give the provider and the public at least 15 days' notice of termination. [42 CF.R. §489.54.] (See "Fraud and Abuse," the last section in this chapter, for more information regarding termination.)

CONDITIONS OF PARTICIPATION

Q.6:18 What are the conditions of participation for the Medicare program?

The Medicare regulations set out the requirements of the statute and additional requirements "considered necessary to ensure the health and safety of patients." [42 C.F.R. §§484.1 *et seq.*] These are known as the conditions of participation, and the regulations specify them in great detail.

An HHA must set forth in writing its organization, the services it furnishes, and its method of operation. Administrative and supervisory functions may not be delegated to another agency, and the HHA must monitor all services not furnished directly.

Q.6:19 What services must an HHA provide?

In order to participate, the HHA must provide part-time or intermittent skilled nursing services and at least one other therapeutic service from among these: physical, speech, or occupational therapy; medical social services; or home health aide services. The services provided must be available on a visiting basis, and in a place of residence used as the patient's home. An HHA must provide at least one qualifying service directly through agency employees but may provide the second qualifying service and any additional service under arrangements with another agency or organization.

If the HHA provides laboratory services, they must be in compliance with the provisions of the Clinical Laboratory Improvement Act. [42 U.S.C. §263a; 42 C.F.R. Part 493.] Most HHAs, since they furnish only the simplest diagnostic tests, are eligible for a waiver under this act.

Q.6:20 What does it mean when services are provided "under arrangements"?

If an HHA must provide certain services to beneficiaries but cannot furnish them itself, it may arrange for another provider to furnish the services. For example, an HHA may arrange with the outpatient department of a hospital or rehabilitation facility to provide services that the HHA cannot provide because the treatment involves use of equipment that cannot be made available to the patient in his or her place of residence.

In such cases, the provider handles all of the details regarding scheduling of treatment, billing, etc., and receives payment directly for the services provided. The secretary does not enter into a provider agreement with the entity providing the services but continues to deal directly with the HHA. However, the HHA is not merely a billing agent for an entity that perhaps is not, in its own right, a Medicare provider. In order for the services to be covered, the HHA must exercise professional responsibility over the arranged services.

Q.6:21 How are services provided under arrangements reimbursed?

The amount charged by the entity that actually supplied the services and was paid by the provider for the services becomes a cost to the provider. This cost is includable in the provider's allowable cost to the extent that the cost is found to be reasonable. Determination of whether it is reasonable is based on the going rate charged for the services within the general community.

Q.6:22 How must an HHA be operated?

A governing body must assume full legal authority and responsibility for operation of the agency. An administrator must organize and direct the ongoing functions of the HHA; maintain links between the governing body, the professional employees, and the staff; employ qualified personnel and ensure adequate staff education and evaluation; ensure the accuracy of public information; and institute an effective budgeting and accounting system.

The HHA must also have a supervising physician or registered nurse (possibly the same person as the administrator) who supervises the skilled nursing and other therapeutic services and who is available at all times during operating hours.

All personnel must coordinate the services they provide in order to support the plan of care. The clinical record or minutes of case conferences must reflect the coordination and communication that occur. A written summary report for each patient must be sent to the attending physician at least every 62 days.

The HHA must have personnel policies as well as personnel records that include information about qualifications and current licensure status.

The HHA must prepare an annual operating budget and a capital expenditure plan.

For personnel under hourly or per-visit contracts or for services provided under arrangements, there must be a written contract specifying the following:

- the services to be furnished;
- the manner in which services will be controlled, coordinated, and evaluated by the primary HHA;
- procedures for submitting clinical and progress notes and for scheduling visits and periodic patient evaluations; and
- procedures for payment for services furnished under the contract. [42 C.F.R. §484.14.]

The contract must also state that patients are accepted for care only by the primary HHA, that personnel must conform to all applicable agency policies, including policies regarding personnel qualifications; and that personnel must participate in development of plans of care.

Q.6:23 What role do professional personnel play in governance of an HHA?

Each year a group of professional personnel, including at least one physician and one registered nurse (preferably a public health nurse) reviews the policies of the HHA. At least one member of the group must be neither an owner nor an employee. The group should review the scope of services offered, admission and discharge policies, medical supervision and plans of care, emergency care, clinical records, personnel qualifications, and the program evaluation. This group should also meet frequently to advise the HHA on professional issues, to participate in the evaluation of the

HHA's program, and to assist the HHA in maintaining links with other health care providers in the community and in the HHA's community information program. [42 C.F.R. §484.16.]

Q.6:24 What are the criteria for acceptance of patients?

Patients are accepted for treatment if it is reasonable to expect that their medical, nursing, and social needs can be met by the HHA. The HHA must develop a detailed plan of care for each patient in consultation with a physician, and this plan must be reviewed at least every 62 days.

Q.6:25 What are the standards for furnishing skilled nursing services?

The HHA must furnish skilled nursing services by or under the supervision of a registered nurse and in accordance with the plan of care. Nursing activities may be performed by either a registered nurse or a licensed practical nurse.

The registered nurse

- makes the initial evaluation visit and regularly re-evaluates the patient's nursing needs;
- initiates the plan of care and necessary revisions;
- furnishes services requiring substantial and specialized nursing skills;
- initiates appropriate preventive and rehabilitative nursing procedures;
- prepares clinical and progress notes;
- coordinates services;
- informs the physician and other personnel of changes in the patient's condition and needs;
- counsels the patient and family in meeting nursing and related needs; and
- participates in inservice programs and supervises and teaches other nursing personnel.

The licensed practical nurse may

- prepare clinical and progress notes;
- assist the physician and registered nurse in performing special-ized procedures;
- prepare equipment and materials for treatments, observing aseptic techniques as required; and
- assist the patient in learning appropriate self-care techniques. [42 C.F.R. §484.30.]

Q.6:26 What are the standards for furnishing therapy services?

Any therapy services furnished by the HHA, either directly or under arrangements, must be given by a qualified therapist or by a qualified therapy assistant under the supervision of a qualified therapist. The therapy must be provided in accordance with the plan of care. The therapist assists the physician in evaluating the patient's level of function and developing the plan of care, prepares clinical and progress notes, advises and consults with the family and other agency personnel, and participates in inservice programs. [42 C.F.R. §484.32.]

Q.6:27 What are the standards for a "qualified therapist" and a "qualified therapy assistant"?

Generally speaking, a qualified therapist, including the occupa-tional or physical therapist, must be a graduate from a program accredited by the appropriate national association and the Ameri-can Medical Association, have two years of appropriate experience, and achieve a satisfactory grade on a proficiency examination con-ducted, approved, or sponsored by the U.S. Public Health Service. Grandfathering provisions apply to physical therapists who met certain criteria regarding membership in professional associations, education, and experience gained prior to 1966 and for physical therapists trained outside the United States.

A qualified therapy assistant must have a combination of education, experience, and certification from accrediting organizations or licensure by the state in which the assistant is practicing. [42 C.F.R. §484.4.]

Q.6:28 What are the standards for furnishing medical social services?

Any medical social services must be furnished by a qualified social worker or a social work assistant under the supervision of a qualified social worker. The social work services must be provided according to the plan of care. The social worker assists the physician and other team members in understanding the significant social and emotional factors related to the patient's health problems, participates in the development of the plan of care, prepares clinical and progress notes, and participates in discharge planning and inservice programs. The social worker also works with the family, uses appropriate community resources, and acts as a consultant to the other agency personnel. [42 C.F.R. §484.34.]

Q.6:29 What are the standards for a "social worker" and a "social worker assistant"?

A social worker must have a master's degree from a school of social work accredited by the Council on Social Work Education and one year of social work experience in a health care setting. A social work assistant must have a bachelor's degree in a field related to social work and have had at least one year of social work experience in a health care setting.

Q.6:30 What are the standards for using the services of home health aides?

Standards for home health aides were upgraded in 1991 in response to problems associated with home health aide services. A home health aide must have successfully completed a state-established or other training program and/or a competency evaluation program or state licensure program. The content of the training programs is rigorous and thorough. An individual who has completed a program but has not furnished home health services for compensation for a continuous period of 24 months since the completion of the program no longer qualifies to deliver home health aide services. [42 C.F.R. §484.36.]

An HHA may offer a training program unless it has been found in violation of applicable regulations within the two years prior to offering the course. For example, it could not offer a home health aide training program if it has permitted an individual who has not passed a training program to furnish home health aide services, has been cited by the state for deficiencies that endanger the health and safety of its patients and has had a temporary management appointed to oversee operations, or has been terminated from participation in the Medicare program.

Q.6:31 What are the training standards for home health aides?

A training program must provide at least 75 hours of classroom training and at least 16 hours of supervised practical training. It must cover many areas of patient care, including communications skills; observation and documentation of patient status; infection control; reading and recording temperature, pulse, and respiration; emergency procedures; personal hygiene and grooming for patients; transfer techniques; and any other task that the HHA wishes the aide to perform. (See *Martin Weissman, Professional Care, Inc., and Israel Cohen v. The Inspector General*, HHS Departmental Appeals Board, Civil Remedies Division, Feb. 14, 1991, Doc. Nos. C-199, 203, in which HHS determined that the owners of a home health agency could no longer participate in Medicare and Medicaid because they had provided homemaker services under Medicaid using the services of untrained and unqualified personal care aides.)

The supervised practical training must occur under the direct supervision of a registered nurse or licensed practical nurse. The practical training must be under the general supervision of a registered nurse with at least two years of nursing experience, at least one year of which must be in the provision of home health care. All training must be documented, and certain competencies must be achieved. A home health aide is not considered to have passed a competency evaluation if the aide has an unsatisfactory rating in more than one of the required areas of training.

An HHA must provide at least 12 hours of inservice training per calendar year to each aide and must complete a performance evaluation of each aide at least every 12 months.

Q.6:32 What sorts of duties may a home health aide perform?

A home health aide is assigned to a particular patient by a registered nurse, who prepares written instructions for patient care. Duties may include personal care, ambulation and exercise, household services essential to health care at home, assistance with medications that the patient normally self-administers, and reporting of changes in the patient's conditions and needs. The aide may also perform simple procedures that constitute an extension of therapy services pursuant to a written plan from a therapist.

If the patient is receiving only home health aide services, a registered nurse must make a supervisory visit to the patient's residence at least every 60 days at a time when the aide is furnishing care. If the patient is receiving skilled nursing care or therapy, a registered nurse or therapist, as appropriate to the care, must make a supervisory visit at least every two weeks.

Q.6:33 What are the necessary qualifications for an administrator of an HHA?

In order to qualify as an administrator of an HHA, a person either must be a licensed physician or a registered nurse or have had training and experience in health service administration and at least one year of supervisory or administrative experience in home health care or a related health field. [42 C.F.R. §484.4.]

Q.6:34 What are the conditions regarding patient rights?

The HHA must provide each patient with written notice of his or her rights in advance of furnishing care or during the initial evaluation visit before initiation of services. The patient may exercise his or her rights, or if the patient has been adjudged incompetent, the patient's family member or guardian may exercise the patient's rights.

In summary, each patient has a right

- to have his or her property treated with respect;
- to voice grievances regarding treatment without fear of reprisal or discrimination;
- to have the HHA investigate complaints;
- to be informed in advance about the care to be furnished, and any changes in that care;
- to participate in the planning of care;
- to receive information regarding advance directives;
- to have clinical records maintained confidentially;
- to be advised, before care is initiated, of the amount of payment expected from Medicare or other sources, and the charges that the individual may have to pay; and
- to be informed about the toll-free HHA hotline, the purpose of which is to receive complaints or questions about local HHAs. [42 C.F.R. §484.10.]

Q.6:35 What are the conditions regarding disclosure of ownership?

The HHA must disclose certain information to the state survey agency at the time of the initial request for certification, for each subsequent survey, and at the time of any change in ownership or management. It must disclose the names and addresses of

- all persons with an ownership or control interest in the HHA;
- each person who is an officer, director, agent, or managing employee; and
- any corporation, association, or other company that is responsible for the management of the HHA and its chief executive officer and chairman of the board of directors. [42 C.F.R. §484.12.]

Q.6:36 What are the conditions regarding clinical records?

The HHA must maintain a clinical record on every patient receiving home health services, including past and current findings, in accordance with accepted professional standards. The record contains the plan of care as well as appropriate identifying information. It also contains the name of the patient's physician; drug, dietary, treatment, and activity orders; signed and dated clinical and progress notes; copies of summary reports sent to the attending physician; and a discharge summary. [42 C.F.R. §484.48.]

Clinical record information must be safeguarded against loss or unauthorized use. Both Medicare and the Joint Commission require written procedures governing the use and removal of records and conditions for release of information, but Medicare explicitly requires the written consent of the patient for release of information not authorized by law.

Q.6:37 How long must an HHA retain its records?

Clinical records must be maintained for five years after the month the cost report to which the records apply is filed with the intermediary unless state law specifies a longer period. The HHA must arrange for retention of the records even if the HHA discontinues its operations. If the patient enters a health care facility, the HHA must send a copy of the home health clinical record with the patient. Although the regulation does not explicitly state this, presumably the HHA could send it directly to the facility.

Q.6:38 Are the clinical records reviewed?

At least quarterly, appropriate health professionals review a sample of clinical records to determine whether established policies are followed in furnishing services directly or under arrangement. Every 62 days, if the patient is still receiving home health services, the clinical record will be reviewed to determine adequacy of the plan of care and appropriateness of continuation of care. [42 C.F.R. §484.52.]

Q.6:39 What are the conditions regarding evaluation of an HHA's program?

The HHA must have written policies requiring an overall evaluation of the agency's total program at least once a year. This evaluation must be performed by a group of professional personnel, HHA staff, and consumers or by professional people outside the agency working in conjunction with consumers. The group reviews overall policies and administrative procedures as well as clinical records and assesses the adequacy of the agency's programs. The group reports to the management of the agency, which is obligated to act upon its findings and recommendations. [42 C.F.R. §484.52.]

Q.6:40 What changes are being discussed with regard to the conditions of participation for home health agencies?

HCFA recently issued a statement expressing its interest in "discussion" of the possibility of revising the conditions of participation. In this statement, HCFA acknowledged that the current conditions do not reflect the mandate in OBRA 1987 to develop outcome-oriented surveys that focus on the quality of care. In particular, the current conditions of participation do not take into account the actual nature of the services being furnished in the home setting. These services, which include parenteral and enteral nutrition, infusion therapy, respiratory therapy, and ventilator services, have become increasingly high-tech. HCFA's recommendations basically propose a more data-driven, quality improvement–based system.

CONDITIONS OF COVERAGE

Q.6:41 What qualifications must a beneficiary meet in order to receive home health services?

In order to receive covered home health services, the beneficiary must meet the following conditions:

- be confined to the home or in an institution that is neither a hospital nor primarily engaged in providing skilled nursing or rehabilitation services;
- be under the care of a physician who is a doctor of medicine, osteopathy, or podiatric medicine; and
- be in need of intermittent skilled nursing care or physical, speech, or occupational therapy. The need for occupational therapy alone will not qualify a beneficiary for home health services initially but will qualify a beneficiary for continued home health services, even after the beneficiary no longer needs nursing care or other kinds of therapy.

Q.6:42 Must the patient pay a copayment or satisfy a deductible in regard to home health services?

No, a beneficiary need not pay a copayment for home health services received. Many of the proposals for health care reform, however, have included a copayment for home health services ranging from 20 to 30 percent. Many home health agencies have expressed concern that a copayment would result in patients refusing home health services because of their inability to pay for them and would also increase the amount of bad debt because of the HHA's inability to collect copayments.

In addition, the beneficiary need not have satisfied the Part A deductible in order to receive home health visits, nor will those visits be counted toward the deductible. Practically speaking, however, a majority of beneficiaries use the home health benefit following a hospitalization or other institutional care, so in fact, their deductible has usually been met.

Q.6:43 How many home health visits may a beneficiary receive?

There is no limit on the number of visits a beneficiary may receive. Services will be provided as long as they are medically necessary.

The Medicare home health benefit is a "sub-acute benefit, not a long-term care custodial benefit. That is, enrollees must have skilled medical needs to be eligible. Home health aide services are covered for beneficiaries who require some skilled nursing or rehabilitation services, but not for those who require only custodial care." [Interim Analysis of Payment Reform for Home Health Services, ProPAC Report, No. C-94-02, March 1, 1994, CCH Medicare and Medicaid Guide, ¶42,119.]

Q.6:44 Must the patient have recently been discharged from a hospital to receive home health services?

No. Under prior law, in order to qualify for home health services, the beneficiary had to be hospitalized for at least three days prior to the receipt of home health services, but this requirement has been eliminated.

Q.6:45 What constitutes a home health service visit?

According to Medicare's basic definition of a home health service visit, "the furnishing of the home health services specified in section 409.40 by a particular health worker on a particular day or a particular time of the day constitutes a home health visit." [42 C.F.R. §409.43.]

The regulation goes on to provide specific examples. If a nurse furnishes several services during a visit (e.g., skilled nursing care and home health aide services), that constitutes only one visit. If, however, both a physical therapist and a visiting nurse furnish services in the home on the same day, or a beneficiary has dressings changed twice in the same day, that constitutes two visits. In addition, if a beneficiary is brought to the hospital for hydrotherapy and while there also receives speech therapy, that also constitutes two visits.

Q.6:46 What is the waiver of liability provision?

Medicare will not pay for services that are "not reasonable and necessary," nor for "custodial care." The ultimate liability for such services falls upon the beneficiary. If, however, the beneficiary did not know that the services would not be covered, Medicare will pay for those services. In addition, if the provider did not know that the services would not be covered, Medicare will pay for the services, but if the provider knew they would not be covered, the provider must pay for the services. [42 C.F.R. §§411.400 *et seq.*]

Q.6:47 How is it determined that a beneficiary knew that services were not covered?

If the beneficiary or someone acting on his or her behalf has been given written notice that the services are not covered, he or she will be considered to have known of the noncoverage. A notice regarding similar or comparable services furnished at an earlier time meets this criterion. The regulation specifies the following example:

> [P]rogram payment may not be made for the treatment of obesity, no matter what form the treatment may take. After the beneficiary who is treated for obesity with dietary control is informed in writing that Medicare will not pay for treatment of obesity, he or she will be presumed to know that there will be no Medicare payment for any form of subsequent treatment of this condition, including use of a combination of exercise, machine treatment, diet, and medication. [42 C.F.R. §411.404]

The notice must have been issued by one of the following parties:

- the PRO, intermediary, or carrier;
- the group responsible for utilization review for the provider that furnished the service; or
- the provider that furnished the service.

Q.6:48 How is it determined that a provider knew that services were not covered?

Similar criteria are applied to the provider as to the beneficiary. The provider is considered to have known that the services were not covered if it received notice from the PRO, intermediary, or carrier; the utilization review committee; the patient's attending physician; or another provider or a practitioner or supplier furnishing the services to the beneficiary informing the provider that the services were no longer covered or that the beneficiary no longer needed covered services.

In addition, if the provider had certain knowledge based on experience or actual or constructive notice of the noncoverage, the provider would be held liable. For example, the provider will be presumed to know the contents of materials received from HCFA, intermediaries, and PROs, such as notices, manuals, bulletins, or other written guidelines.

When a provider has made reasonable efforts to ensure that its Medicare coverage decisions are in line with program policies and procedures and has in the past demonstrated an ability to make appropriate coverage decisions, it will be presumed that the provider did not have knowledge of noncoverage.

Medicare has stated specific numeric criteria for determining whether an HHA had notice. Intermediaries collect statistics to determine whether denial rates exceed 2.5 percent for HHAs for medical necessity denials and 2.5 percent for technical denials. The HHA will be re-evaluated at least every three months and may be re-evaluated sooner if the HHA experiences drastic fluctuations in rates.

Q.6:49 What must an HHA do if noncovered services have already been paid for?

The HHA will have to refund the payment unless it can show that it did not know and could not reasonably have been expected to know Medicare would not pay for the service or that it informed the beneficiary the services may not be paid for and the beneficiary signed a statement agreeing to pay for the service. If proper notice was given, the HHA may receive a "waiver" of liability for the refund.

Q.6:50 What type of notice must be given for an HHA to receive a waiver of liability?

The notice must be in writing and use approved notice language, citing the particular services for which payment is likely to be denied and why the HHA believes the services will be denied. This notice will not be acceptable if the HHA routinely gives it to all beneficiaries and if it does not state strongly enough that payment may be denied.

CONDITIONS OF PAYMENT

Q.6:51 What are the general conditions for payment by Medicare?

In order for services to be paid for, they must meet the following criteria:

- They must be covered services and be furnished by a provider qualified to have payment made for those services at the time they were furnished.
- They must have been furnished to an individual who was eligible to receive them at the time they were furnished.
- They must be certified by a physician and recertified as necessary.
- The HHA or the beneficiary, as appropriate, must file a proper claim, with sufficient information to determine whether payment is in fact due and the amount of that payment. [42 C.F.R. §§424.1 *et seq.*]

Q.6:52 What are the physician certification requirements?

The physician is the driving force in the provision of health care services furnished by providers. Therefore, as a condition for Medicare payment, a physician must certify the necessity of the services and, in some instances recertify the continued need for those services. [42 C.F.R. §§424.10 *et seq.*]

Q.6:53 What are the responsibilities of a provider regarding physician certification requirements?

The provider must obtain the required certification and recertification statements, keep them on file for verification by the intermediary, and certify on the billing form that the statements have been obtained and are on file. The statements may be in any form that meets the needs of the provider as long as it permits verification. For example, they may be entered on forms, notes, or records that a physician signs for other purposes or on a separate form for certification purposes only. While certification statements need not be on a special form, there must be a separate signed statement for each certification or recertification.

Q.6:54 What are the specific physician certification requirements for home health services?

Each certification must state that the individual needs intermittent skilled nursing care or physical, speech, or occupational therapy; that home health services are required because the individual is confined to the home except when receiving outpatient services; and that a plan for furnishing the services has been established and periodically reviewed by a physician.

Q.6:55 What must a recertification contain?

Each recertification must state that the need for services is continuing and estimate how much longer the services will be required. If the beneficiary has a need for occupational therapy, this need may be the basis for continuing services that were initiated because the individual needed skilled nursing care or physical or speech therapy.

Q.6:56 Under what circumstances may a physician not be involved in the certification-recertification process?

If a physician has a significant ownership interest in or a significant financial or contractual relationship with an HHA, that physician may neither certify or recertify the need for services, nor establish or review a plan of treatment for that HHA.

A significant ownership interest is defined as a direct or indirect ownership interest of 5 percent or more in the capital, stock, or profits of the HHA or an ownership interest of 5 percent or more in any mortgage, deed of trust, note, or other obligation that is secured by the agency if that interest equals 5 percent or more of the agency's assets.

A physician is considered to have a significant financial or contractual arrangement with an HHA if he or she receives any compensation as an officer or director of the HHA. An uncompensated officer or director may perform certification functions for the HHA. In addition, if the physician has direct or indirect business transactions with the HHA that, in any fiscal year, amount to more than $25,000 or 5 percent of the HHA's operating expenses, whichever is less, the physician may not certify the need for services. Business transactions include contracts, agreements, purchase orders, or leases to obtain services, supplies, equipment, space, and salaried employment.

These restrictions on physician certification do not apply if the HHA involved is a sole community HHA or is operated by a federal, state, or local governmental authority.

Q.6:57 When are the certification and recertification obtained?

The initial certification of need for home health services must be obtained at the time the plan of treatment is established, or as soon afterwards as possible, and must be signed by the physician who established the plan. The recertification must be obtained at least every two months, preferably when the plan is reviewed. It must be signed by the physician who reviews the plan.

Q.6:58 What type of certification is necessary for reimbursement for home medical equipment?

All orders for HME must be made pursuant to a physician's order. These orders must be written and must contain the folowing information:

- the patient's medical diagnosis, by ICD-9-CM code, and the patient's prognosis;
- the initial date on which the equipment should be delivered and an estimate of how many months the patient will need the equipment;
- the justification, from a medical standpoint, for the equipment;
- a description of the equipment and its related supplies; and
- administrative information, including insurance information, and the physician's signature and date.

Q.6:59 What additional documentation is required for certain types of HME?

Certain items need an additional type of certification known as a certificate of medical necessity (CMN). This is an additional form that the physician must complete in detail regarding the need for the equipment. The list of items for which a CMN is required changes periodically but generally includes items that have been subject to overutilization or other forms of abuse. For most items requiring a CMN, it is not necessary to also have a written order, as the information would be redundant.

Suppliers often have difficulty obtaining the completed form from the physicians, as it adds to their paperwork burden. It is crucial, however, that no individual other than the physician complete the full CMN. Neither supplier personnel nor HHA personnel may complete the CMN, although they may provide certain specific information prescribed by the law. In addition, there are varying policies regarding the use of a faxed CMN, which is easier to obtain, and regional carriers processing HME claims have distinct views on its acceptability.

Q.6:60 What is the method for reimbursing home health care costs?

Costs are reimbursed based upon the reasonable costs incurred to provide the services, calculated retrospectively. [42 C.F.R. Part 413.] Actual reimbursement is the lower of these two figures: the reasonable costs and the HHA's customary charges for the services provided. Reimbursement is calculated on a per-visit basis using time records submitted to the agency by the personnel making the visits.

Assuming that the reasonable cost is lower than the HHA's customary charges, which it almost always is, Medicare reimburses 100 percent of the reasonable cost of the services furnished by or under arrangements made by the HHA. The determination of reasonable costs takes into account both the direct and indirect costs of providing services to Medicare beneficiaries. Indirect costs include items such as depreciation, interest, bad debts, educational costs, and compensation of owners.

Q.6:61 How is the amount of reasonable costs determined?

Reimbursement is made on a retrospective basis for costs actually incurred during the previous year. The HHA submits a cost report detailing the costs related to the services furnished to Medicare beneficiaries. The HHA may receive interim payments in order to minimize cash flow problems, and the agency and Medicare settle any discrepancies in overall reimbursement after the cost report is submitted.

Q.6:62 What is the cost allocation process?

In preparing the cost report, indirect costs are allocated in accordance with the services the HHA has provided as a means of determining its actual costs per visit. This is referred to as the step-down process. The indirect costs are allocated based upon the direct costs of each direct service even if that service is not a covered home health benefit. In order to avoid the allocation of indirect costs to a noncovered and therefore nonreimbursable service, the HHA must first assign its indirect costs to reimbursable or nonreimbursable services. This process is known as discrete costing.

Q.6:63 What is the cost apportionment process?

Once the actual costs have been determined, they must be apportioned between Medicare and non-Medicare patients, as it is a primary principle of cost reimbursement that no part of the costs of services provided to non-Medicare patients must be borne by the program, nor may costs of services provided to Medicare patients be borne by other patients. The costs of all visits of a certain type (e.g., occupational therapy visits) are aggregated, including both Medicare and non-Medicare, and the reimbursement due is determined by calculating the percentage of the costs associated with the services to Medicare beneficiaries.

Q.6:64 What limitations are placed on reimbursement for home health services?

Reimbursement is not unlimited, and reimbursable costs may not exceed the costs estimated by HCFA to be necessary for the efficient delivery of needed health services. Thus, HCFA sets "cost limits" indicating the maximum amount Medicare will reimburse for each type of service an HHA provides. The cost limits are applied, however, in the aggregate—to the total agency costs. Thus, an HHA may exceed the limit for one or two types of services it provided but have costs lower than the limit for other services; as long as the total costs do not exceed the total amount of the limits, the HHA would receive reimbursement for all of its costs.

The calculation of cost limits includes labor-related and non-labor-related costs. Currently, the cost limits are set at 112 percent of the mean per-visit cost for all free-standing agencies [42 U.S.C. §1395x(v)(1)(L)(i)], and are recalculated annually by HCFA and published in the *Federal Register*. Health reform proposals working their way through Congress are recommending lowering the cost limits to, for example, 100 percent of the median, a reduction that would be devastating to home health agencies.

Q.6:65 What if a provider's costs exceed the cost limits set by HCFA?

The regulations provide a means for requesting an exception to the cost limits. As HCFA estimates that 38 percent of HHAs are at or over the cost limits, such requests are fairly routine. An adjustment is made to the cost limits only to the extent the costs are reasonable, attributable to the circumstances specified, separately identified by the provider, and verified by the intermediary. The specific exceptions that apply to an HHA are these:

- *Atypical services.* Either the items provided by the HHA are atypical in nature and scope or the patients have special needs and require atypical items.
- *Extraordinary circumstances.* Unusual occurrences such as flood, strikes, fire, and earthquake caused the provider to incur higher costs.
- *Unusual labor costs.* The percentage of labor costs varies more than 10 percent from that included in the calculation of the limits.

Providers requesting an exception to the cost limits may be reviewed operationally by HCFA. HCFA may then recommend changes to improve the efficiency and economy of the HHA's operations. Any future exceptions would be contingent on the HHA's implementation of the recommendations.

In addition, there are limited circumstances in which the HHA may charge the beneficiary for items that are more expensive than those determined by Medicare to be necessary for the efficient delivery of needed health care. The HHA must identify such charges for the beneficiary and must request the intermediary to validate these charges before charging the beneficiary for them.

Q.6:66 How can the Medicare program verify the costs of services provided to HHAs under contract with other entities?

Medicare requires all contracts between a provider and a subcontractor to allow program representatives access to the subcontractor's contract, books, documents, and records until the end of the fourth year after the services are furnished. If such a clause is not included in a contract, no payment for the services furnished under that contract will be made. [42 C.F.R. §§420.300 *et seq.*] The requirement applies to contracts representing services, but not supplies or equipment, that have a cost or value of $10,000 or more over a 12-month period.

Thus, if an HHA subcontracts with another HHA or a physical therapy group to provide professional services and the services meet the monetary and time criteria, the contract must contain the required clause. Or if the HHA is the subcontractor, the HHA must ensure that the contracting entity has included this clause in the agreement.

HHS will request access to records only under certain circumstances:

- it has reason to believe the costs claimed for the services provided by the subcontractor are excessive or inappropriate;
- there is insufficient information to judge the appropriateness of the costs;
- there is a written accusation with suitable evidence against the provider or subcontractor of kickbacks, bribes, rebates, or other illegal activity; or
- evidence shows that the provider did not disclose a related organization.

Any request by HHS must be in writing and contain the following elements:

- reasonable identification of the materials requested;
- identification of the contract or subcontract in question;
- the reason that access is necessary;
- the statutory and regulatory authority for the access;
- identification of the individuals who will be visiting the HHA to obtain access, the time and date of the scheduled visit, and the name of an HHS representative to contact if questions arise.

Once HHS makes its request, the subcontractor will have 30 days from the date of the request to make the records available. If the subcontractor believes that the request does not meet the criteria listed above, it may notify the requestor of the problem within 20 days. Once the requestor responds, the HHA has 20 days to provide the information during regular business hours.

If HHS requests the HHA to photocopy records, HHS will pay for such costs, but if the HHA photocopies them independently, the HHA must pay for the copies and no Medicare reimbursement is available for the costs. HHS may examine originals if it prefers. If the subcontractor refuses to make records available, HHS may initiate legal action against the subcontractor.

Because all agreements with subcontractors must contain an "access to records" clause, a sample provision follows.

> *Access to Records.* Provider shall take all necessary steps to ensure full and complete access to any and all records, equipment, and supplies necessary for the performance of the services specified in this Agreement. Provider shall keep confidential all information relating to the facilities and beneficiaries it serves.
>
> If under the Medicare/Medicaid Acts or regulations promulgated thereunder the Provider should be deemed to be a subcontractor under 42 U.S.C. §1395x(v)(1)(I), Provider shall make available to the Secretary of the Department of

Health and Human Services or of the Comptroller General, or to its duly authorized representatives, a copy of this Agreement and such books, documents, and records of the Provider as are necessary to certify the nature and extent of the services performed hereunder. If Provider carries out any of the duties of this Agreement through a subcontract, having a value or cost of $10,000 or more over a twelve (12) month period with an organization within the meaning of 42 C.F.R. §405.427, such subcontract shall contain a clause to the effect that, until the expiration of four (4) years after the furnishing of services, the related organization shall make available to the Secretary, Comptroller General, or to any of their authorized representatives the subcontract, the books, documents and records of the related organization as necessary to verify the nature and extent of costs incurred pursuant to this subcontract.

Q.6:67 What is prospective payment?

In 1983, the Medicare program changed the method of reimbursement for hospital inpatient costs from a retrospective, reasonable cost–based system to a prospective system, known as the prospective payment system (PPS). Under PPS, hospitals receive for each type of case a payment determined by the diagnosis-related group (DRG) into which the case falls.

The intent of Congress in establishing PPS for hospital payments was to push hospitals to operate more efficiently, for under PPS a hospital could easily lose money if it used resources ineffectively. If the hospital uses fewer resources than allowed for a particular DRG, the hospital still receives the full payment allotted for that case and retains the extra amount. If, however, the hospital's costs exceeded the payment allowed for a particular DRG, the hospital would have to absorb the extra costs.

Other benefits of this method of payment are the simplicity of administration and related reduction of administrative burdens on hospitals and more accurate identification of methods in which certain services could be provided at a lower cost. As a practical matter, the hospital administration and medical staff work more closely together to achieve the efficiencies possible under the system. Congress provided for annual review of the system by the Prospective Payment Assessment Commission (ProPAC).

This commission has recently issued a report presenting its "background analysis" of the Medicare home health agency benefit. The report confirms that the secretary of health and human services is developing a program to modify the current home health agency benefit or to develop a prospective payment system for HHA reimbursement. In its report, ProPAC did not make any substantive recommendations regarding prospective payment but indicated that it will respond directly to the secretary's proposed payment revisions when they are published. [Interim Analysis of Payment Reform for Home Health Services, ProPAC Report, No. C-94-02, March 1, 1994, CCH Medicare and Medicaid Guide, ¶42,119.]

The home health industry, however, seems to be involved in the process of reviewing on its own the possibility of a prospective payment system for home health services. Recent demonstration studies based upon a per-episode methodology have not proven positive, and currently other studies are underway using the per-visit methodology.

FRAUD AND ABUSE

Q.6:68 What are the "fraud and abuse" laws?

The fraud and abuse laws are a section of the Medicare Act designed to curb practices that in the early years of the Medicare program led to overutilization of services under the program. The first set of Medicare fraud and abuse laws was enacted in 1977, and the laws have evolved and become much more sophisticated since then.

Q.6:69 What specific actions are prohibited under the fraud and abuse laws?

The Medicare and Medicaid statutes generally prohibit the following types of activity:

- The submission of false claims, for the purpose of obtaining payment or benefits. Omission of information for this purpose is also prohibited.
- The provision of false information or material misrepresentation of facts to obtain or maintain certification as a Medicare participating home health agency.
- Conversion of any payment from the program to a use other than for use of the person on whose behalf the payment was made.
- Solicitation, receipt, offer, or payment of any remuneration (including kickback, bribe, or rebate), in return for referral of Medicare or Medicaid patients or in return for recommending or arranging for the purchase, lease, or ordering of any Medicare- or Medicaid-related service. This prohibition is known as the "antikickback statute." [42 U.S.C. §1320a-7b.]

Q.6:70 What types of activities might be suspected of involving false claims?

In order for an HHA to be criminally liable under the false claims statute, the action must have been "knowing and willful." Simply submitting an incorrect claim, either with wrong information about the services provided or about the individual to whom the services were provided, is not grounds for prosecution under the statute. Obviously, if the HHA intended to defraud the program and submitted the false claim as a means to that end, it would be construed as a "knowing and willful" submission. Under the statute, however, the simple act of submitting a claim in which the HHA knows there is incorrect information, even if it had no intent to defraud the program, would open the HHA up to charges of fraud and abuse.

False claims may include the following:

- submitting a claim for services that were never rendered to the beneficiary or that the HHA knew were not medically necessary for the beneficiary;

- submitting a claim for services that were actually rendered and were medically necessary but providing false information to substantiate the claim;
- receiving Medicare benefits that are rightfully due to another HHA;
- submitting duplicate bills, such as submitting two claims to Medicare for the same service or one claim to Medicare and another claim to the beneficiary for the same service;
- submitting claims for services provided by practitioners who have been excluded from participation in the programs or who are unlicensed; and
- submitting claims at higher prices for Medicare and Medicaid patients than for other patients.

Q.6:71 What types of actions does the antikickback statute prohibit?

As with the prohibitions on false claims, in order to be in violation of the antikickback statute, the HHA must have performed an action "knowingly and willfully." The statute is written so broadly that the HHA can violate the statute through an action without knowing that the action was *illegal*. As long as the action itself was intentional, such as payment to a physician for referral of a patient, there need not have been any separate intent to defraud the program.

In general, the following types of activity are prohibited:

- soliciting or receiving any type of remuneration; or
- offering or paying any type of remuneration in return
  —for referring any individual to a person for the furnishing, or arranging for the furnishing, of any item or service for which some payment may be made by Medicare or Medicaid; or
  —for purchasing, leasing, ordering, or arranging for or recommending such actions for any good, facility, service, or

item for which some payment may be made by Medicare or Medicaid.

The prohibition covers both parties involved in a transaction: the one who offers and the one who receives remuneration.

Q.6:72 What types of remuneration are prohibited under the statute?

The prohibited remuneration may be in the form of kickbacks, bribes, and rebates, which are the most obvious types of incentives given for referrals or inducements. In addition, the statute prohibits remuneration in any other form if it is for the purposes named above. Such prohibited remuneration may be "direct or indirect," "overt or covert," or "in cash or in kind."

Q.6:73 How have provider actions been scrutinized under case law?

Case law interpreting the statute has applied these principles as broadly as possible, to cover many types of payment scenarios. For example, even if the remuneration was, indeed, made for a lawful purpose, such as to compensate for services rendered to the provider by another provider, if only one of the purposes of the remuneration was unlawful, such as to induce referrals in addition to compensating for services rendered, the conduct violates the statute. [See *United States v. Greber*, 760 F.2d 68 (3rd Cir. 1985).]

In another case, HHS determined that a provider can violate the statute even if an offer or payment is based not upon an explicit agreement to refer, but upon an offer or payment made with the intent to exercise influence over the professional judgment of the providers as an inducement to refer. [See *Inspector General v. Hanlester Network, et al.*, Dkt. No. C-448, Dec. No. CR181 (March 10, 1992).] The following types of conduct by the providers were suspect and ultimately determined to be unlawful and should be avoided:

- The providers offered physicians investments in the laboratories to encourage those physicians to refer business to the laboratories.
- The providers made it clear to the physicians that the ultimate success of the laboratories was dependent upon their referrals.
- The providers offered the physicians high rates of return if certain referral volumes were attained and discouraged them from referring their business to other laboratories.

Q.6:74 Are there any types of payments that will not be suspect under the antikickback statute?

Yes, there are four types of payments that are set out in the statute as exceptions to the rule:

1. Discounts or other reductions in services that an HHA may obtain in the regular course of its business, as long as the discounts are disclosed to Medicare on the cost report or otherwise and are passed on to Medicare. Obviously, Medicare wants to encourage providers to provide their services at the lowest possible charge, which may be accomplished through obtaining services from their suppliers at a discount. If, however, the HHA receives a 30 percent discount from a supplier, it cannot bill Medicare at the full price, even if that price is at or below limitations on costs or charges, and keep the discount for itself. The "discount exception" would not apply if the HHA does not pass the discount on to Medicare.
2. Payments to employees under a bona fide employment relationship established for the purpose of providing covered items or services.
3. Payments to a group purchasing agent, as long as the vendor and agent have a written agreement that specifies a fixed amount or fixed percentage of sales as the agent's fee and the agent discloses the amount of vendor payments

made to Medicare providers upon request by the secretary
of health and human services. Again, Medicare encourages
efficient program operation, and as long as an agent
provides services for a fixed fee, one that is not related
directly or indirectly to the volume of sales, the transaction
will be protected under this exception.
4. Payments made that fall into one of the "safe harbors,"
which are types of arrangements that the secretary of health
and human services has determined will not violate the
statute. [42 U.S.C. §1320a-7b.]

Q.6:75 What other type of guidance is available to help an HHA avoid engaging in fraudulent or abusive practices?

The Medicare program has issued several fraud alerts, in which
the program targets specific practices and describes the characteristics of practices which will draw scrutiny by the Office of Inspector
General.

The first fraud alert in 1989 described some of the features of "joint
ventures" that might be suspicious. Basically, joint ventures with
physicians are viewed as an attempt to capture their referrals rather
than to simply raise start-up capital. The OIG looks at the investors
and their role and treatment by the venture, the business structure
of the venture, and the financing and distribution of profits.

For example, a venture that offered physicians and investment
interests in proportion to their expected volume of referrals, that
tracks the source of referrals and distributes the information to
investors, or that requires investors to divest their ownership interest if they cease to practice in the service area would be suspect.
Likewise, a joint venture that appeared to be only a "shell," with all
of the day-to-day business carried on separately by the two parties
in their particular businesses, might have a questionable business
structure. Finally, if physicians invest only a nominal amount and
are paid extraordinary returns, the venture would be suspect on
these grounds.

A second fraud alert issued in 1991 prohibited providers from
routinely waiving the beneficiary's copayment and/or deductible

amounts. Basically, the program views this as a misrepresentation of the charge for the service. For example, if the charge is $100, the copayment should be $20, with Medicare paying the remaining $80. If, however, the copayment is waived, the charge should now be $80, and Medicare should pay only $64 (i.e., 80 percent of the actual charge of $80).

The OIG is concerned about the effect of waivers on utilization of program services. If a provider routinely waives a copayment, the beneficiary will likely be induced to purchase items and services from that provider, possibly leading to overutilization of the services because they are free. Although currently there are no copayments for HHA services, it is likely that such copayments will become a feature of HHA reimbursement, and this prohibition will have greater relevance. Even absent such copayment, however, this serves as an example of the type of activity that will trigger scrutiny by the OIG for fraud and abuse.

Q.6:76 What sorts of arrangements have been specifically protected under the fraud and abuse laws?

Under the Medicare and Medicaid Patient and Program Protection Act (MMPPPA), the secretary of health and human services was specifically directed to publish regulations describing payment practices that would not be considered to violate the antikickback provisions. [42 C.F.R. §§1001 et seq.] If a provider complies with these regulations, any payment arrangements will be "safe," which explains the use of the term "safe harbor" to describe these practices.

No violation will have occurred if a payment comes from one of the safe harbors described in general terms below:

- An investment interest in a large, publicly traded entity.
- An investment in a smaller entity, as long as no more than 40 percent of the investment interests held during the previous fiscal year or 12-month period is held by investors who are in a position to make or influence referrals to, furnish items or services to, or otherwise generate business for the entity and less

than 40 percent of the entity's gross revenues comes from referrals from investors.

- Lease of space, as long as the lease agreement
    —is set out in writing and signed by the parties;
    —clearly identifies the leased property;
    —specifies the anticipated times (if not full time) and nature of use;
    —is for at least one year so that it cannot be adjusted during the year to reflect referral volume; and
    —reflects fair market value.

- Lease of equipment, with the same conditions as described above for the lease of space.

- Personal services and management contracts, with the same conditions as above for the lease of space and equipment, except that the second requirement addresses the services to be provided rather than property. In addition, this safe harbor requires that services performed under the agreement do not involve counseling or promotion of a business arrangement or other activity that violates any state or federal law. Thus, contracts with marketing or sales personnel who are not employees but rather independent contractors must be drafted to meet the requirements of this safe harbor so as to ensure that the individuals are not marketing illegal arrangements.

- Sale of a practice that will be completed within a year and where the selling practitioner will not be in a position to refer buiness to or generate business for the purchaser.

- Referral service for generating and managing referrals for physician services, as long as the referral service does not exclude any qualified physician from participating; charges the same fee to all physicians and the fee is reasonably related to the cost of running the service; imposes no requirements on the manner in which the physician provides services; and tells individuals using the referral service how physicians are selected, whether the physicians have paid a fee to participate in the service, how the service is related to the physicians it refers, and how the service excludes physicians from participating.

- Warranties, including those given by a manufacturer for the products of others as well as their own, as long as the parties report any price reduction of the item that was obtained as part of the warranty.
- Discount, as long as the discount is a reduction in the amount the seller charges for a good or service and not just a rebate, a giveaway of goods or services, a coupon, or another in-kind form of remuneration. The discount must also appear on the sales invoice or statement and in the buyer's cost report or claim. Thus, an HHA may not offer extra services or coupons for items as an inducement for referrals, either directly to the patient or to a physician for referral of a patient.
- Bona fide employment relationship, where the employer pays the employee for providing covered items or services. This safe harbor uses the IRS definition of employee and protects remuneration to part-time employees but not to independent contractors.
- Group purchasing agent, as long as the agent or organization does not wholly own the entities furnishing health care services, or own the entities through a subsidiary relationship. The agent must have a written agreement with each purchasing entity specifying that the agent will receive no more than 3 percent of the purchase price of the goods or services provided by any given vendor, or if the fee is not fixed at 3 percent, specifying the amount the agent will be paid. The agent must disclose annually to each participating provider of health care goods or services the amount received from each vendor in return for purchases made by that provider.

The OIG has recently issued proposed clarifications of the safe harbor rules relating to investment interests, referral services, discounts, rental agreements, and personal services contracts. These clarifications would result in greater scrutiny by the OIG of arrangements under these provisions. [See 59 *Federal Register* 37202 (July 21, 1994).]

Additional safe harbors relating to the provision of services under managed care plans have been developed. One of these relates to the price reductions providers offer to health plans in order to obtain access to the plan's patients and increase the provider's volume. This safe harbor requires that if the plan is under contract with HCFA or a state agency, the provider must not claim payment except as approved by HCFA and may not shift its costs to any other payers. In addition, the safe harbor requires that agreements between the health plan and the contract health provider be for not less than one year and specify in advance the covered items and services and the obligations to file claims. Finally, it requires that the provider maintain a stable fee schedule throughout the term of the agreement and bill according to the fee schedule.

Q.6:77 What criminal penalties are imposed for violation of the fraud and abuse laws?

Violation of the statutes addressing false claims and illegal remuneration may result in fines of up to $25,000 and imprisonment of up to five years. In addition, other federal criminal statutes provide sanctions that may be applicable in fraud and abuse actions. These include the following:

- Mail Fraud, 18 U.S.C. §1341, which prohibits use of the U.S. Postal Service in the furtherance of any "scheme or artifice to defraud." Violation is a felony and punishable by up to $10,000 in fines and five years' imprisonment.
- Criminal False Claims Act, 18 U.S.C. §287, which prohibits the filing of a claim with any government employee with the knowledge that it is false, fictitious, or fraudulent. Violation is a felony, and punishable by up to $10,000 in fines and five years' imprisonment.

Q.6:78 What civil penalties are imposed for violation of the fraud and abuse laws?

Certain civil penalties, known as civil money penalties, may be imposed upon program participants for presentation of false claims of certain kinds. [42 U.S.C. 1320a-7a; 42 C.F.R. §§1003.100 *et seq.*] An HHA could be liable for such civil penalties for the following actions:

- presenting a claim for an item or service that it knew or should have known was not provided as claimed or was fraudulent;
- presenting a claim for an item or service furnished during a period in which the HHA was excluded from participation in the program;
- seeking payment in violation of the terms of an assignment agreement, a limitation on charges or payments, or a requirement not to charge in excess of the amount permitted under Medicare;
- misusing certain words, letters, symbols, and emblems associated with the program, such as "Social Security," "Medicare," or "Health Care Financing Administration."

If it is determined that more than one person was responsible for a violation, each person may be held liable for the penalty. Penalties range from $2,000 for each item or service improperly made, to $5,000 for each misuse of program symbols, to $15,000 for each person involved in the false claim. In addition, a person, or the HHA itself, may be assessed an amount up to twice the amount actually claimed, not just paid, for each item or service that was the basis for the underlying penalty. The person may also be excluded from participation in both Medicare and Medicaid as a result of the penalty, unless the state waives the exclusion.

In determining the amount of the penalty, the OIG will consider the following:

- the nature of the claim and the circumstances under which it was presented;
- the degree of culpability of the person submitting the claim;
- the history of prior offenses;
- the financial condition of the offender; and
- in the case of misuse of department symbols, the nature of the communication, the degree to which any misrepresentation

may have been mitigated by a disclaimer of association with the government, and the history of prior similar offenses.

Q.6:79 Can an HHA be assessed a civil money penalty based upon the same violations that resulted in a criminal conviction?

Yes. One case specifically looked at the question of whether a subsequent civil money penalty would violate the double jeopardy clause of the United States Constitution and determined that it could, because the civil penalty amounted to a punishment unrelated to the goal of compensating the program. [*United States v. Halper*, 109 S. Ct. 1892 (1989).] Subsequent cases, however, have held that the double jeopardy clause was not violated because the purpose of the penalties was compensatory rather than punitive. [See *United States v. Pani*, 717 F. Supp. 1013 (S.D. N.Y. 1989); *Manocchio v. Kusserow*, 961 F. 2d 1539 (11th Cir. 1992).]

Q.6:80 What other sanctions may be brought against a person who files false claims?

Under the federal False Claims Act, the attorney general or a private person may bring a civil action on behalf of the government against any person who has obtained or attempted to obtain money from the government by making a false statement or otherwise filing a false claim. [31 U.S.C. §3729.] In addition, the HHA's provider agreement may be terminated if the HHA engages in fraudulent or abusive conduct. [42 U.S.C. §1395cc(b)(2).]

Q.6:81 What is the exclusion provision and how is it implemented?

The OIG has the authority to exclude individuals and entities from participating in federal and state health care programs. [42

U.S.C. §1320a-7.] The Medicare and Medicaid Patient and Program Protection Act of 1987 regulations [57 *Federal Register* 3298 (Jan. 29, 1992)], specify certain types of activities that give the power to the OIG to exclude a provider. There are two types of exclusions: mandatory, which must be for a minimum of five years, and permissive (or discretionary), which is usually for a period of three years.

The OIG may exclude an HHA from receiving payment for services to Medicare or Medicaid beneficiaries using the mandatory exclusion provisions if the HHA is convicted of a criminal offense related to the delivery of an item or service under Medicare or Medicaid or any other state health care program that receives federal funds. Exclusion may also result if the provider is guilty of patient abuse or neglect. [42 U.S.C. §1320a-7a.]

In one recent case, a home health agency was excluded under the mandatory exclusion provisions from participation in Medicare and Medicaid for 15 years for providing homemaker services using untrained and unqualified personal care aides. [*Martin Weissman, Professional Care, Inc., and Israel Cohen v. The Inspector General*, HHS Departmental Appeals Board, Civil Remedies Division, Feb. 14, 1991, Doc. Nos. C-199, 203, 205.] In this case, the owners were convicted of two felonies and a misdemeanor related to the operation of their home health agency. First, they were convicted of grand larceny for filing fraudulent claims with the state Medicaid program, seeking payment for homemaker services rendered by untrained and unqualified personal care aides. As a result of the conduct, the Medicaid program paid the owners approximately $1.8 million to which they were not entitled. Second, they were convicted of falsifying business records as a result of the actions of one of the managerial employees of the agency. The misdemeanor charge was for conspiracy related to the owners' decisions to alter the personnel records after the fact to conceal the failure to comply with Medicaid regulations and to escape possible liability for overpayment.

The Health and Human Services Departmental Appeals Board's analysis exemplifies the steps in applying a mandatory exclusion. First, the board found that the owners were, in fact, convicted of a criminal offense "related to the delivery of an item or service" under the Medicaid program. The fraudulent conduct comprised both the provision of homemaker services and the falsifying of the related records, and the board expressly stated,

> [T]he Medicaid program requires that agencies providing home health care services meet record-keeping requirements to document that its aides are trained, healthy, and otherwise qualified. The record-keeping requirements are an integral part of a regulatory scheme designed to ensure that Medicaid recipients receive competent home health care services. It is apparent from this regulatory scheme that the Medicaid program did not view its requirements to document the qualifications of personal care aides as being separable from its objective to provide competent home health care services to Medicaid recipients. . .

In addition, the board found that the conduct was related to the delivery of an item or service under Medicare or Medicaid because the "victim" of the crime was, in fact, the program. The "adverse impact" of the crime on the program "is not tangential or ephemeral," but rather the "activity damaged program integrity, resulted in a monetary loss to the program, and breached [the owners'] duty to program recipients." Thus, the board strongly believed that the conduct in this case was so clearly fraudulent in relation to the program that the mandatory exclusions were applicable.

The next step in the exclusion process is to determine the length of the exclusion appropriate in any given case. The minimum period under the mandatory exclusion provision is five years, and according to the regulations at 42 C.F.R. §1001.128(a)(3), the "ultimate issue to be determined . . . is whether the exclusion is reasonable." In arriving at the 15-year exclusion for the owners of the HHA, the board considered the purpose of the exclusion process, remarking that the removal of an untrustworthy provider serves to shut off a "potential avenue for causing harm to the program or to its beneficiaries or recipients" as well as "deterring other providers" from causing such harm. The board acknowledged that the exclusion would likely have an adverse financial impact on the HHA but emphasized that "exclusion is not punitive if it reasonably serves the law's remedial objective, even if the exclusion has a severe financial impact on the individual or entity against whom it is imposed."

The board went on to make the following conclusions of law, which led it to believe that a substantial exclusion was appropriate:

- The owners were convicted of serious offenses, and their attempt to evade exclusion by shifting responsibility to low-level employees was not persuasive. The board found that the management of the HHA knew about the bookkeeping changes and "made a decision at the management level to agree to this activity so that the corporation would not have to return any money overpaid to it by Medicaid."

- The owners committed the criminal activities over a lengthy period of time.

- The criminal offenses underlying the convictions resulted in substantial financial damage (at least $1,000,000) to the Medicaid program and seriously compromised the integrity of the program.

- The criminal offenses underlying the convictions endangered the health and safety of Medicaid recipients.

- The above offenses alone were sufficient to warrant a 15-year exclusion, but in addition the board found evidence of widespread misconduct spanning a number of years. For example, if inservice training documents, reference letters, and physical forms were missing from the files, the spouses of the owners would generate the forms for the file. They also changed test scores when the owners learned that the passing grade was higher than the grades some of the aides had attained on their tests. The owners not only "agreed" to the falsification efforts but sometimes participated in them.

- The HHA had prior administrative sanctions for noncompliance with documentation requirements and other substantial deficiencies.

- The owners' "persistent misconduct in the face of administrative sanctions and their efforts to deceive government auditors" constituted a "serious aggravating factor," and the fact that they operated a business that served the community by delivering home health services did not rise to the level of a "mitigating circumstance" that could lessen the exclusion period.

The board concluded its opinion by reiterating the facts of the case, showing the owners' pattern of misconduct and untrustworthiness justified the 15-year exclusion. The Board further emphasized the ancillary effect of deterring other individuals from engaging in such conduct, given that "home care is a large and fast growing industry," and therefore "is easy prey for unscrupulous providers." The exclusion was at least, in part, intended to "send the message that home health care providers who engage in this kind of behavior can expect to incur substantial exclusion from participation in Medicare and Medicaid."

Q.6:82 For what types of activities may the Office of Inspector General exclude a provider under the permissive exclusion regulations?

The OIG has broad discretion to exclude a provider under the permissive exclusion provisions. [42 C.F.R. §§1001.201 *et seq.*] Any of the following activities or events may trigger scrutiny:

- Conviction under federal or state law of a criminal offense for fraud, theft, embezzlement, breach of fiduciary responsibility, or other financial misconduct in connection with the delivery of any health care service.
- Conviction under federal or state law of interference with or obstruction of an investigation into a criminal offense in connection with a health care program.
- Conviction under federal or state law of a criminal offense relating to the unlawful manufacture, distribution, prescription, or dispensing of a controlled substance.
- Having a license to provide health care revoked or suspended or otherwise losing a license for reasons bearing on professional competency or performance or on financial integrity.

- Suspension, exclusion, or other sanctions on participation in a federal or state health program for reasons related to professional competence or performance or on financial integrity.
- Submitting excessive claims or furnishing unnecessary or substandard items and services.
- Failure of health maintenance organizations, competitive medical plans, and primary case management systems participating in Medicare to provide medically necessary items and services where that failure has adversely affected or has a substantial likelihood of adversely affecting covered individuals.
- Where false or improper claims for items and services have been submitted under Medicare or a state health care program.
- Where a significant shareholder or investor, officer or director, partner, agent, or managing employee of an entity has been convicted of a program-related criminal offense and has had a civil monetary penalty imposed against him or her or has been excluded from participation in Medicare or state health programs.
- Where an individual or entity is involved in a kickback arrangement prohibited under the criminal antikickback statute.
- Failure to disclose ownership or control information as required by the program.
- Failure to provide payment information.
- Failure to provide immediate access upon reasonable request to surveyors to determine compliance with conditions of participation.

Q.6:83 What if the above violations do not involve Medicare or Medicaid beneficiaries but relate only to private-pay patients?

Entities and individuals can be excluded from the Medicare or Medicaid programs for violations that relate only to patients covered by private insurance. Exclusion can occur when an entity or individual furnishes items or services substantially in excess of a patient's needs or of a quality that fails to meet professionally recognized standards of health care, regardless of the payer source. [42 C.F.R. §1001.101(a)(2).]

Q.6:84 If an HHA provides noncovered items and services, would the provision of these items and services be considered excessive?

According to the regulations [42 C.F.R. §1001.101(a)(2)], providing noncovered services would not be considered provision of excessive services, if the items and services were requested by the patient, and the HHA informed the patient that they were not medically necessary and were not covered by Medicare or Medicaid. Medicare requires an HHA to inform the patient in advance in such situations [42 C.F.R. §§484.10(e)(1) and (2)], and the HHA should document in the patient's chart that it has informed the patient adequately.

Q.6:85 What types of cited deficiencies under other administrative programs put an HHA at risk for exclusion?

HHAs are subject to surveys for Medicare certification purposes, for state licensure purposes, and for accreditation by the Joint Commission. Sometimes these agencies find alleged violations of state, federal, or professional standards in an HHA's operations.

As part of determining whether the violations are serious and coming up with a way to remedy them, the agency and the HHA enter into an agreement (or settlement), in which they detail the method the HHA will use to fix the problems. It is possible that any deficiencies cited as part of the survey and/or the settlement document could be used as the basis of an exclusion under the argument that the HHA failed to provide care according to professionally and administratively established standards.

Therefore, any agreement that an HHA enters into in settlement of a licensure, reimbursement, or coverage dispute must be carefully worded so that the terms cannot be used as the basis for an exclusion action at a later date. At a minimum, the agreement should state that payment under the terms of the settlement is not an admission of wrongful action.

Q.6:86 What are "prohibition against physician self-referral" provisions?

The Omnibus Reconciliation Act (OBRA) of 1993 amended existing law, 42 U.S.C. §1395nn(a), known as the "Stark Act," after Representative Fortney "Pete" Stark (D-Calif.), who authored the law. The Stark Act prohibited physicians from referring Medicare patients to laboratories with which they have a financial relationship, either an ownership or investment interest or a compensation arrangement. The prohibition also applies if an immediate family member of the physician has the ownership or investment interest or the compensation relationship. The law recognizes that physicians are the primary initiators of utilization of health care services and attempts to curb overutilization and abuse by removing any incentives to refer patients for unnecessary services.

OBRA 93, known as "Stark II," contained specific prohibitions against "self-referral" to additional designated health services for Medicare and Medicaid beneficiaries. Thus, beginning January 1, 1995, under these prohibitions, physicians may not refer to the following types of entities if they have a financial relationship with the entity:

- clinical laboratories;
- home health services;
- physical and occupational therapy services;
- radiology or other diagnostic services;
- radiation therapy services;
- furnishing medical equipment;
- furnishing parenteral and enteral nutrients, equipment, and supplies;
- furnishing prosthetics, orthotics, and prosthetic devices;

- outpatient and prescription drugs; and
- inpatient and outpatient hospital services.

Q.6:87 What is meant by a "financial relationship"?

A financial relationship is defined as an ownership interest or a compensation arrangement. An ownership interest is defined in the law as any equity or debt interest, except for ownership of investment securities in large publicly held companies. A provider of home health services with a physician owner must furnish the secretary of health and human services with information concerning the ownership arrangements.

A compensation arrangement is any arrangement involving remuneration between a physician or immediate family member and an entity to which the physician refers. Thus, any relationship of either of these types between an HHA and a physician will be suspect under Stark II.

Q.6:88 What is meant by a "referral"?

The definition of referral is very broad. It includes, obviously, a direct request or order by a physician for the provision of home health services. In addition, a referral includes a request for consultation with a second physician who then orders home health services or performs or supervises them. Such a transaction would have been prohibited had the first physician done it directly, and thus the law does not allow the physician to make that referral through another individual.

Of special interest to home health agencies is the aspect of the definition of referral that addresses a plan of care. A request for or establishment of a plan of care by a physician that includes home health services rises to the level of a referral. Thus, a physician cannot develop a plan of care for a patient that includes home health services provided by an entity with which the physician has a financial relationship.

Q.6:89 What are the penalties for making prohibited referrals?

Medicare will not pay for any services provided in violation of the Stark laws, and payment received from other sources must be refunded. In addition, civil monetary penalties of up to $15,000 for each service furnished illegally may apply. The provider may be excluded from participation in the program, and may be assessed fines of up to $10,000 per day in which violations occurred, and up to $100,000 for creating a scheme to "circumvent" the law.

Q.6:90 What types of ownership interests by a physician in an HHA may fall into the category of exceptions to the prohibition against self-referrals?

Several exceptions are defined in the law. First, the exception discussed above at question 6:87 applies to ownership interests in a large publicly held company, (i.e., a company that has stockholder equity in excess of $75,000,000 and whose stock is available to the general public through a national or regional stock exchange).

In addition, an ownership exception applies to home health services provided by a rural provider, i.e., one whose services are mostly provided to individuals residing in a rural area. This provision protects access to home health services—and of course all designated health services—in rural areas. Further, if a general hospital provides home health services, a physician with an ownership interest in that hospital may still refer for home health services if the physician has privileges at the hospital and the ownership interest is in the hospital itself rather than a division of the hospital or subsidiary.

Q.6:91 What types of compensation arrangements between a physician and an HHA may fall into the category of exceptions to the prohibition against self-referrals?

The statute provides that such an arrangement does not include the rental of office space or equipment, a bona fide employment relationship, or remuneration not connected with the provision of health services. For example, if the HHA and physician have a rental agreement for the lease of office space, that lease will not be in violation of the self-referral prohibition as long as that lease meets the following qualifications:

- The lease must be in writing and signed by the parties and be specific about the premises covered under the lease.
- The space leased must not exceed the amount reasonable and necessary to fulfill the legitimate business purpose of the lease and must be used exclusively by the lessee (except for common areas, which may be used pro rata).
- The term of the lease must be at least one year.
- The rental payments must be consistent with fair market value, must be set out in advance, and must not be determined in a manner that takes into account the volume or value of any referrals.
- The lease must be commercially reasonable even absent any referrals by the parties.

In addition, a bona fide employment arrangement will be acceptable as long as the arrangement is

- for identifiable services;
- consistent with fair market value and not based on the volume or value of any referrals made by the physician; and
- commercially reasonable, even without any referrals.

Other exceptions include personal service arrangements, based upon the personal services safe harbor, and services for which remuneration does not relate to the provision of designated health services. For example, if a physician is hired as the medical director of an HHA, the physician may continue to refer patients to the HHA or to develop plans of care including the HHA's services as long as the remuneration for his or her duties as medical director are not based upon the provision of the HHA's services to patients.

Physicians and HHAs may also engage in one-time transactions, such as the sale of real or personal property, as long as the transactions are commercially reasonable and the compensation is consistent with fair market value and unrelated to referrals. Thus, for example, an HHA may sell a physician one of its investment properties or vehicles as long as the sale meets the above requirements.

Q.6:92 What is the relationship between the ownership provisions of the Stark II provisions and the physician certification requirements?

The ownership provisions of these two sets of requirements are clearly in conflict in several ways. Before discussing these differences, it should be noted that until these conflicts are resolved, HHAs should abide by the most stringent of the requirements of each provision, even if a specific provision or exemption exists in the other provision in a relaxed form.

First, the certification regulations specify that a physician may not refer to a home health agency in which he or she has a significant financial or ownership interest, which is defined as 5 percent or more of certain defined assets and expenses of the HHA. The Stark II law, on the other hand, prohibits a referral to an HHA in which the physician has "a financial interest," which is defined, in part, as "an ownership interest." The interest need not be 5 percent, and thus *any* ownership interest will trigger the prohibition against a referral.

A second form of "significant financial interest" under the certification scheme is a compensation or contractual arrangement that provides the physician more than $25,000 per year. The Stark II law, however, prohibits referrals where *any* compensation arrangement exists unless it meets one of the statutory exceptions. For example, if the lease exception applies, the HHA could have a lease transaction with the physician even if it was more than $25,000.

Another difference is the prohibition by Stark II against referral even if the financial interest is with the spouse or other family member of the physician, whereas the certification provisions have no such prohibition (i.e., the family member could hold the interest and the physician could still refer to the HHA). The certification provisions also are not affected by the safe harbors that insulate the HHA against the antikickback provisions. So, for example, if an HHA pays a physician a salary, that physician cannot refer to the HHA, whereas under the employee safe harbor the physician could continue to refer to the HHA.

Finally, one notable difference between the two sets of requirements is that the certification regulations provide no civil or criminal penalties. The only sanction is denial of coverage of items or services that the physician certified or reviewed. The Stark II law provides for specific penalties levied against the HHA of up to $15,000 for each service supplied.

7

Patient Care Issues

Once the home health agency has established itself as a viable business entity, hired the right people to deliver the care and run the business, and created a place for itself in the market, all that really matters is that the agency deliver care in a manner that serves its patients well. Patients must be treated properly, and the relationship between agency and patient, once established, must be pursued in a certain manner. Agency personnel must obtain valid consent for performing certain procedures and must comply with new federal mandates regarding the nature of that consent. Finally, unlike a hospital admission, the relationship between a home health agency and its patients may continue for a long period of time, and the agency must carefully define the parameters of that relationship so that patients are clear about the services to be provided.

ABUSE AND NEGLECT

Q.7:1 Are HHA personnel required to report to any authority if they believe a patient is being abused?

Yes. Most states have enacted laws requiring individuals who have professional contact with an individual to report to local law enforcement authorities if they have observed the individual being subjected to abuse, neglect, self-neglect, or exploitation or have other reason to believe such kinds of treatment have occurred. [See Md. Code Ann. Family Law Article §14-302 (dealing with abuse of adults) and Md. Code Ann. Family Law Article §§5-701 *et seq.* (dealing with child abuse and neglect).]

Professionals who are required to make such reports include physicians, nurses, therapists, police officers, social workers, and other human service workers. In addition, any other individual who suspects such treatment may make a report and obtain the protection of the law but is not required to do so. If, for example, a neighbor suspected that an individual was being abused or neglected and mentioned this to the HHA employee on one of the visits to the home, the HHA worker would be obligated to mention this either to authorities or to the HHA administration, but the neighbor would have no duty to report.

Q.7:2 Is the HHA liable if its personnel fail to report abuse or neglect?

The HHA could be held liable for failure to report a reportable event. Under the doctrine of *respondeat superior*, the employer can be held liable for the acts of the employees if those acts were done in the course of the employment. By the same token, the employer may be held liable for omissions of the employee if those omissions are related to the employment. In fact, however, if the HHA properly trained the employee regarding the duty to report and the employee did not report abuse to either the HHA or to law enforcement authorities, the HHA would most likely not be viewed as liable for the failure.

Many of the laws regarding reporting require a health care practitioner acting as a staff member of an institution to report the incident to the administration of the institution. Thus, if the nurse reported the incident to the HHA administrator or other management personnel, the HHA would be required to act upon the report in accordance with the specific procedures in the particular state law. If the HHA did not act upon the information, the agency and not the employee would be liable.

Q.7:3 Can the HHA be held liable for reporting suspected abuse or neglect if the allegations turn out to be untrue?

No. Generally, the same statutes that require certain persons to report suspected abuse or neglect also provide immunity from civil liability for making a report as well as from any participation in the related investigation or judicial proceedings.

Q.7:4 What types of information should be reported to authorities?

The report should be as comprehensive as possible so that the authorities, or possibly the court if the individual refuses to accept social services directly, may fashion the best relief for the patient. It should contain at least the following minimal information, but it will certainly be accepted even if it has less information than that listed:

- name, age, and home address of the individual;
- name and home address of the person responsible for the care of the individual;
- nature of the disability or incapacity of the individual;
- nature and extent of the abuse, neglect, self-neglect, or exploitation of the individual;
- any information that would help determine the cause of the abuse or neglect and the person responsible for it.

The appropriate authorities will use the information in the report to conduct an investigation into the abuse and take steps to protect the individual.

Q.7:5 Must an HHA disclose a patient's medical records during an investigation of alleged abuse or neglect?

In most states, the HHA will be required to disclose the patient's medical records if they are needed by the local law enforcement agency or social services department in furthering the investigation into the abuse or neglect.

CONSENT

Q.7:6 What is the basic principle of consent?

Historically, a health care provider must obtain consent before performing any procedure on a patient. If the provider performs the procedure without the required consent, the provider can be civilly liable to the patient for invasion of privacy as well as criminally liable to the patient for an assault or battery.

Q.7:7 Who may legally give consent for treatment?

Any competent adult may give consent for treatment for him- or herself. A competent adult may also give consent for treatment of a minor for whom he or she has legal responsibility. For example, if the adult is the child's parent or legal guardian or is caring for the child and has a power of attorney authorizing him or her to obtain medical care for the child during the period of custody, that adult may consent to any medical treatment for the child. The law presumes that a patient is competent to provide consent unless the patient gives clear indication of incompetence.

In an emergency situation, no actual consent is necessary. Consent to treatment in an emergency is presumed, as long as health care providers limit the scope of treatment to procedures that address the immediate medical needs. For example, emergency treatment for cardiac arrest would include cardiopulmonary resuscitation, intravenous administration of appropriate medications, and perhaps a tracheotomy but would clearly not include bypass surgery to alleviate the arteriosclerosis that may have caused the cardiac arrest.

Q.7:8 What form must the consent take?

The consent may take different forms:

- Oral discussion and agreement. The physician explains the procedures and the positive and negative effects, and the patient verbally consents to the procedures. In this situation, the health care provider should note prominently in the medical record that the patient was informed regarding the procedure and that the patient verbally consented. If possible, the provider should have the patient sign or initial the medical record.

- Implied consent. Although express or explicit consent is preferred, the law will sometimes imply consent if sufficient indications exist. For example, if the patient expresses complete submission to the provider's professional judgment, this may be interpreted as a general authorization for treatment. The treatment, however, should be appropriate for the condition for which the patient initially sought treatment. Once the original condition is treated, the implied consent will not cover further treatment for unrelated conditions. In emergency situations, of course, consent is implied, even if the emergency occurs during a procedure for which the patient consented and the emergency requires treatment outside the first procedure.
- Written consent. In most situations, the health care provider will have a consent form for the patient to sign. This form should allow the patient and provider to specifically designate the procedures or treatment for which the consent is valid. A written consent which generally authorizes the provider to treat the patient, without specifying what the patient is being treated for, may be held invalid because of its ambiguity.

Q.7:9 What additional steps must a provider take regarding consent?

As discussed above in question 7:7, the law clearly requires the provider to obtain consent to treat a patient either from the patient him- or herself or from an individual legally authorized to consent on his or her behalf. A simple "yes, sir," however, is not sufficient. The required consent can be described as somewhat of a "consent plus," given after the patient has received a reasonably understandable explanation of the treatment. In other words, the consent must constitute "informed consent."

The rationale behind requiring informed consent is that if the patient or the patient's representative is unaware of the full implications of the treatment, the consent does not really reflect a choice. Informed consent represents a legal acknowledgment of the principle that a patient has the right to self-determination (this right is the basis of the Patient Self-Determination Act) and must have access to all relevant information in order to exercise control over his or her own body.

Q.7:10 What are the standards for determining whether a patient's consent was informed?

There are two primary and possibly conflicting standards for determining the nature and scope of the informed consent for any particular patient. The traditional standard relates to the health care provider's opinion as to what the patient is able to comprehend and absorb, balancing the provider's assessment of the state of the patient's physical and mental health against the nature of the possible negative consequences of the treatment and the likelihood of their occurrence.

The more modern standard measures the consent from the patient's point of view, with the physician responding to what the patient wants or needs to know rather than what the physician thinks the patient needs to know. This determination may be made by the caregivers in response to express questions by the patient or by engaging the patient in a discussion that reveals the patient's needs for information. In some jurisdictions, the standard for informed consent may require disclosure of the risks and benefits of other treatment alternatives, and many consent forms include specific sections for alternatives to the recommended or selected treatment.

Below is a sample form for obtaining consent. Note that it contains a release of claims, which the user may or may not wish to include (the release also may or may not be legally effective, depending on the circumstances and the jurisdiction).

CONSENT TO TREATMENT

Date: _____
Time: _____

I have been fully informed by my health care provider, _____, of the advantages

and the possible risks and consequences of the treatment for
_____, which include
_____
_____
_____.

Given this information, I hereby consent to such treatment and
agree to hold _____ harmless for any claims,
demands, or suits for damages from any injury or complications of
any kind, except those arising from negligence, that may result from
the treatment I have accepted.

[Signature of patient] or

[Signature and relationship of person legally authorized to consent
for patient]

Q.7:11 What procedures are available if consent cannot be obtained from the patient?

If an HHA has determined that the patient is not competent to
give consent, the HHA should check to see if the patient has
executed an advance directive. This is a form that allows the patient
to make his or her wishes known regarding health care. If no such
document has been executed or can be found, the HHA should
determine whether another individual with authority is available to
consent on the patient's behalf. This individual is known as a
"surrogate decisionmaker." A discussion of both of these modes of
health care decisionmaking follows.

ADVANCE DIRECTIVES

Q.7:12 What is an advance directive?

An advance directive is an instrument created by an individual
that gives information about the type of medical treatment the
individual wishes to have or not to have if he or she ever becomes
unable to make decisions for him- or herself.

Generally, such instruments should be written, dated, and signed by two witnesses but some states allow health care providers to honor oral directives if they are properly executed. Such an oral directive shall have the same effect as a written directive if the statement is made in the presence of the attending physician, and one witness, and documented as part of the individual's medical record. [See Ohio Revised Code Ann. §127.505 (Baldwin 1995); Md. Code Annotated, Health General Article §§5-601 *et seq.*; Fla. Stat. Ann. §§765.101 *et seq.* (West 1994).]

Q.7:13 Who may legally serve as a witness to the creation of an advance directive?

Any individual who is competent and who does not have a financial interest in the property of the person executing the document may serve as a witness. Some states allow staff of the health care facility treating the patient to serve as witnesses, while other states do not allow such persons to serve as witnesses.

Q.7:14 What are the most common types of advance directives?

The two common types of advance directives are the living will and the durable power of attorney for health care. It is advised that individuals execute both types, as they have different functions.

Q.7:15 What does a durable power of attorney for health care accomplish?

In a durable power of attorney for health care, the individual names another person to make medical decisions for him or her if the individual becomes unable to make them on his or her own behalf. The person named is called the "agent" or "proxy." The agent may be anyone the individual selects, the most common choice being the spouse, a child, or a close friend.

In this instrument, the individual specifies what sort of treatment he or she would like provided or withheld under certain types of circumstances. The key word is "durable," which indicates to the subsequent reader of the document that the author intended for it to survive any disability. Thus, physicians and nurses involved with an HHA patient who has executed such a document should have no doubt about when to follow its directives, unless it appears that the document was coerced.

Q.7:16 What does a living will accomplish?

A living will is generally created for the same purposes as a durable power of attorney for health care, except that it is usually applicable to situations where the individual who executed it is terminally ill. The contents usually refer to the withholding or furnishing of treatment to a terminally ill individual. Unlike the case of the durable power of attorney, the instructions in the living will are acted upon without the intervention of an agent. Thus, it is important that an HHA be aware of the existence of a living will and understand its terms.

Most states have living will forms available for their citizens. While an individual may execute a living will in any form, it is preferable to use the state form so that caregivers, who will be familiar with the form, will feel comfortable following its provisions.

Q.7:17 What is the Patient Self-Determination Act?

The Patient Self-Determination Act (PSDA), which was part of the Omnibus Budget Reconciliation Act of 1990, includes specific requirements for health care providers regarding the right of patients to make health care decisions. The PSDA conditions Medicare and Medicaid participation on the provider's development of policies that address the means by which patients can make their own health care decisions, including the execution of advance directives.

Q.7:18 To what types of providers does the PSDA apply?

Hospitals, skilled nursing facilities, hospices, and home health agencies participating in the Medicare and Medicaid programs are required to develop policies of the type set out in the act.

Q.7:19 What sorts of activities are mandated by the PSDA?

The requirements of the PSDA involve administrative activities. The PSDA does not specify any particular content for an advance directive. To comply with the administrative responsibilities of the act, an HHA must do the following:

- Maintain written policies and procedures for all adults receiving medical care through the provider or organization concerning their rights under state law to make decisions concerning their medical care, accept or refuse medical or surgical treatment, and formulate, at the individual's option, an advance directive or not.
- Provide written information to all adults on these policies, including the HHA's policies respecting the implementation of these rights. The information must be given in writing before the individual receives care.
- Document in the individual's medical record whether or not the individual has executed an advance directive.
- Not condition the provision of care or otherwise discriminate against an individual based on whether or not that individual has executed an advance directive.
- Ensure compliance with requirements of state law (statutory and through case law) regarding advance directives.
- Provide for the education of staff and the community on issues concerning advance directives.

Q.7:20 Can an advance directive be revoked?

Yes. Virtually all state laws regarding advance directives provide that an advance directive in any form can be revoked. In order to ensure that it is appropriately revoked, the individual should put any change or cancellation in writing, sign and date it, and give copies to his or her doctor and family and any other person who might still have a copy of the original. Some states allow an advance directive to be changed or revoked orally.

Ideally, revocation is done before any need for services arises, but if services are already being rendered and the individual is still competent, the individual should notify his or her doctor, family, etc. Even if the individual merely states directly to the physician his or her wishes and does not put them in writing, the oral expression of wishes will generally carry more weight than an older written document. The individual should insist that the physician enter a note into the chart noting the changes and should sign and date the note.

Q.7:21 How does the PSDA interact with state law as regards advance directives and surrogate decisionmaking?

The PSDA grants to individuals the rights that are provided in state law. It does not provide any new rights to patients, nor infringe upon any existing rights. The PSDA formally requires providers to inform patients of these rights and to assist patients in effecting their own advance directive if they so desire. The specific provisions in any documents created by the patients, however, are governed exclusively by state law.

Q.7:22 Does an HHA have to comply with the provisions of an advance directive?

Most states address situations in which a patient has an advance directive but the provider, either for religious or moral reasons, is unable to comply with the requests of the patient. In this type of situation, an HHA must inform the patient that its personnel cannot carry out the instructions and that the patient may obtain another health care provider. The HHA must assist the patient in obtaining another provider. If, however, this process of switching would take too long and the patient might die before the transfer could occur, the provider must comply with the advance directive.

Q.7:23 Where should information about advance directives be kept?

An HHA should document in a patient's medical record that he or she has executed an advance directive. Any HHA personnel should review the advance directive carefully and document that they have reviewed it. If possible, the HHA personnel should discuss the terms of the advance directive with the patient and any caregivers to be certain that the caregivers understand its terms and the patient's wishes.

Q.7:24 What legal actions may be taken for an incompetent patient if an advance directive does not exist?

If an incompetent patient has not executed an advance directive, the HHA may look to either a surrogate decisionmaker or a guardian if one has been appointed. In an emergency situation, an HHA would be required to seek or provide medical treatment without appropriate consent to the point where the patient was stabilized. At that point, the HHA should attempt to reach a surrogate decisionmaker or ascertain whether a guardian has been appointed.

SURROGATE DECISIONMAKING

Q.7:25 What is a surrogate decisionmaker?

A surrogate decisionmaker is an individual who stands in the stead of a legally disabled or incompetent individual for the purpose of making decisions for that person. These decisions may range from financial and daily living decisions to decisions regarding medical care for the individual. Many states have enacted statutes that allow for surrogates to make decisions for disabled individuals. In all cases, however, the HHA must ensure that the individual meets the state's enumerated criteria for "incompetence" or "disability" before attempting to identify and work with a surrogate.

The main advantage of having surrogates defined by statute is that the health care providers need not institute court proceedings in order to obtain consent for treatment of an incompetent or disabled individual. Health care providers simply need to locate a surrogate in one of the appropriate groups and evoke his or her opinion as to the best course of action for the patient and obtain his or her consent to that treatment.

Maryland's new Health Care Decisions Act has provisions for surrogate decisionmaking. It is one of the most detailed and liberal of such statutes and is becoming a model for other states as they address these problems through legislation. Thus, Maryland's law is discussed below as an example. [See Md. Ann. Code Health General Article §§5-601 *et seq.*; Florida Statutes Ann. §§765.101 *et seq.*]

Q.7:26 What standards should the surrogate decisionmaker use and what factors should be considered in making a decision on behalf of a disabled individual?

The authorized surrogate decisionmaker should base his or her decisions on the wishes of the patient. If those wishes are unknown or unclear to the surrogate or others involved in the care of the patient, the decisions should be based on the patient's best interests. Factors to be considered include the patient's

- current diagnosis and prognosis with and without the proposed treatment;
- expressed wishes regarding the provision of or withholding or withdrawal of the proposed treatment or similar treatments, including expressed concerns about the effects of the treatment on family or intimate friends;
- religious and moral beliefs and personal values; and
- indications through behavior and attitudes regarding the type of treatment at issue and medical treatment in general.

The Maryland statute specifically prohibits the surrogate from considering any pre-existing, long-term mental or physical disability the patient has or the patient's economic position.

Q.7:27 Who may be a surrogate decisionmaker?

The potential surrogates are listed in the statute in order of priority. Health care providers must attempt to consult individuals in the higher class of surrogates first, moving down the list only if the members of the higher class are unavailable. The order is as follows:

- guardian, if one has been appointed;
- patient's spouse;
- adult child of the patient;
- parent of the patient;
- adult brother or sister of the patient;
- legally competent friend or relative.

In order to qualify as a surrogate, a friend or relative must execute an affidavit stating his or her relationship to the disabled person and listing specific facts and circumstances demonstrating that he or she has maintained regular contact with the patient so as to be familiar with the patient's activities, health, and personal beliefs. [See also Florida Statutes Ann. §765.204.]

Q.7:28 How does a health care provider determine if surrogates in a particular class are unavailable?

For purposes of contacting a surrogate in the next priority class, a health care provider can conclude, as a legal matter, that a particular surrogate is "unavailable" if

- the health care provider has made reasonable inquiry and has either not identified any surrogate decisionmaker in the appropriate class or, if one has been identified, has not been able to locate that individual;

- the surrogate decisionmaker has not responded in a timely manner, considering the specific health care needs of the disabled individual, to attempts at contact by the health care provider (the contact should be made in writing, if possible, but a verbal attempt is legally sufficient); or
- the surrogate decisionmaker is incapacitated or otherwise unwilling to make decisions concerning health care for the individual.

"DO NOT RESUSCITATE" ORDERS

Q.7:29 What is a "do not resuscitate" order?

A "do not resuscitate" (DNR) order is a written medical order prepared by the attending physician that documents instructions by an adult patient or, if the patient is incompetent, the patient's appointed or statutory surrogate or an otherwise appointed proxy. This document is also known as a cardiopulmonary resuscitation (CPR) directive. [Wyoming Statutes, Public Health and Safety, Living Will, Art. 2.] It instructs caregivers or others present at the time a patient may experience cardiac or respiratory arrest that cardiopulmonary resuscitation is to be withheld. [See, *e.g.*, Civil Rights §765.101.] Any adult who has the decisional capacity to provide informed consent to or refusal of medical treatment or has been authorized through an advance directive to make decisions for an incapacitated person may execute a DNR order.

Q.7:30 What form must a DNR order take and what information should be included?

The requirements vary from state to state. In Wyoming, for example, in order to be valid and honored by medical personnel, a DNR order must be executed on a form issued by the state department of health. It should contain the following types of information regarding the person who is the subject of the order:

- the person's name, date of birth, sex, eye and hair color, and race or ethnic background;
- the name, address, and telephone number of the person's attending physician and, if applicable, the name of a hospice program in which the person is enrolled;
- the person's signature or mark or the signature or mark of a person authorized to execute such a directive on the behalf of the person;
- the date on which the DNR order was signed;
- the specific information concerning the administration of the DNR order, countersigned by the person's attending physician.

Q.7:31 If no DNR order has been executed, can medical personnel still withhold CPR?

No. In the absence of a DNR order or CPR directive, a person's consent to cardiopulmonary resuscitation should be presumed. In addition, if there is any doubt as to the authenticity of an order that exists, perhaps because of the date on which it was issued, medical personnel must administer CPR.

It is prudent for HHA personnel to discuss DNR orders with the patient at various times during the course of treatment. If one has not been executed at the beginning of treatment, the nurse should mention it as a possibility. Once it is executed, the nurse should remind the patient of its existence and verify that the patient intends for the order to remain in effect.

Q.7:32 Must medical personnel, including HHA personnel, comply with a DNR order?

Yes, if that order is apparent and immediately available. Generally, any person who complies with such an order that appears to be valid and therefore does not attempt to resuscitate a patient will be immune from civil or criminal liability or any sort of regulatory sanction for complying with the order. Any health care provider who is unable to comply with a DNR order, for moral or other reasons, should take steps to transfer the patient to another provider before the need for compliance with the order arises. Thus, if an HHA nurse knows that a patient has executed a DNR order, and it is posted in the home, that nurse should request a transfer to another assignment, ensuring meanwhile that the patient receives care from another HHA nurse.

Q.7:33 May a DNR order be revoked?

Yes. A DNR order may be revoked at any time, either by the individual to whom it applies or by a surrogate authorized to act on that individual's behalf. Immediately upon revocation, the HHA personnel should note in the medical record that the DNR order has been revoked and should remove it from the location in which it had been displayed.

GUARDIANSHIP OF DISABLED OR INCOMPETENT PERSONS

Q.7:34 What is a guardian?

A guardian is an individual appointed by the court to direct the affairs of a disabled person. This disabled person is often referred to as the "ward." State courts have the authority to superintend the care of disabled persons, hence the familiar term "ward of the state." In the exercise of its authority, the state court may appoint an appropriate individual to act as the disabled person's guardian. The guardianship may be as broad or as narrowly defined as is necessary to provide for the demonstrated need of the disabled individual.

Q.7:35 What is the difference between a surrogate decisionmaker and a guardian?

A surrogate decisionmaker is determined by statute and chosen by a caregiver or other involved individual at the time of a need for a decision. In contrast, a guardian is generally appointed by the court in advance of any need for a particular decision, but rather in response to the disabled person's overall need for help.

In addition, a surrogate is authorized to make health care decisions only, whereas a guardian is appointed for the purpose of making general and day-to-day decisions about the person's welfare, including but not limited to health care.

Q.7:36 What two types of guardian may be appointed by the court?

If a person is "disabled," this means that he or she is unable to manage personal affairs and property effectively. The cause for the inability to manage property may be either physical or mental disability, senility or another type of mental weakness, disease, habitual drunkenness, or addiction to drugs. [Maryland Rule 70.] If such conditions exist, the court may appoint a guardian to protect the person or the person's property, or both. A guardian of the property may be appointed if the disability stems from compulsory hospitalization, confinement, or disappearance.

Both types of guardianship have serious implications—they both essentially deprive an individual of basic rights of decisionmaking and management of his or her own affairs. Appointing a guardian of the property is usually more straightforward. The evidence is usually clear as to whether the individual can manage property: If accounts are maintained and bills are paid and personal property is in order, generally the court will not appoint a guardian of the property. The individual will be presumed in control of his own property absent any indication of material waste. If, however, the court determines that the individual needs a guardian of the person, a guardian of the property will most likely be appointed as well. An HHA and its various types of personnel will most likely be involved in the guardianship of the person.

Q.7:37 What grounds must exist for appointment of a guardian of the person?

A guardian of the person is an individual appointed by the court to direct the care of a disabled person. A guardian of the person is appointed according to the following standard:

[T]he court determines from clear and convincing evidence that a person lacks sufficient understanding or capacity to make or communicate responsible decisions concerning his person, including provisions for health care, food, clothing or shelter, because of any mental disability, senility, other mental weakness, disease, habitual drunkenness, or addiction to drugs, and that no less restrictive form of intervention is available which is consistent with the person's welfare and safety. [Md. Code Ann. Estates and Trusts Article §13-705.]

Q.7:38 What is the effect on a disabled person of having a guardian appointed?

In order to appoint a guardian of the person, the court must first adjudicate that person "disabled." This determination, however, is not the same as declaring the person legally "incompetent," which is, for example, the standard of review for committing a person to a mental institution. Thus, in most states, an adjudication of "disability" for the purpose of guardianship of a person is insufficient basis for admitting someone to a mental institution.

In addition, such an adjudication may not be the basis for modifying any civil right of the disabled person, including any right related to civil service rank, appointment, licensure, permit, privilege, or benefit under any law. For example, a person who cannot, as a matter of daily living, take proper care of him- or herself or who cannot be trusted to make appropriate decisions regarding his or her personal affairs may still be able to drive or even hold a job. Such a person may need a guardian but could continue to work as a licensed barber, for example, as long as he or she was able to perform the necessary tasks.

Q.7:39 What are some of the duties and rights of a guardian of the person?

State statutes vary in their enumeration of the duties and rights of guardians of the person. They are generally the same rights and duties that a parent has with regard to an unemancipated minor child, including but not limited to the following:

- The duty to provide for the care, comfort, and maintenance of the disabled person. This duty encompasses providing for social interaction as well as for education and training, if appropriate, for the disabled individual.
- The duty to take reasonable care of the personal property of the disabled person, including furniture, clothing, and vehicles. This duty also encompasses the right to initiate protective proceedings against personal property if necessary.
- The right to compel any other person to perform a duty to support the disabled person and to compel the guardian of the property to furnish adequate support, including using the funds in the estate to pay third persons for care and maintenance of the disabled person.
- The right to custody of the disabled person and to establish that person's place of residence, with or without court authorization as appropriate, according to the particular state's law.
- The duty to file an annual report with the court indicating the disabled person's place of residence and health status, the plan for the person's future maintenance, and the status of the guardian.
- The power to give consent or approval, as required by state law, for medical or other professional care or the withholding or withdrawal of such care, except that the court must authorize a guardian's consent to any medical treatment that involves a substantial risk to the disabled person's life. [See Md. Code Ann. Estates and Trusts Article §13-708.]

Q.7:40 Is a guardian of the person liable to third parties for acts committed by the disabled person?

No, the guardian of the person is specifically exempt from liability for acts committed by the disabled person. Thus, if a patient of an

HHA is under a guardianship of the person and that patient injures HHA personnel or steals HHA property, the guardian may not be held liable for those actions. The HHA may sue the estate for financial redress and obtain funds from the guardian of the property, but it may not sue the guardian of the person individually for damages.

Q.7:41 What is the procedure for obtaining a guardianship?

The first step in obtaining a guardianship is the filing of the petition with the appropriate court. Any "interested" person may file such a petition. Interested persons include the guardian, the heirs, the disabled person, any governmental agency paying benefits to the disabled person, and any person named by the court as having a substantial interest in the appointment of a guardian.

Practically speaking, any individual who observes the disabled person and identifies the need for a guardian may petition the court. Often the petitioner is the social services agency providing for the disabled person; the social security office, which might notice an irregularity in the cashing of checks; or a hospital where the disabled person has been admitted.

Q.7:42 What information must be in the petition?

The petition must be signed and verified by the petitioner and contain the following information:

- The name, age, sex, and address of the alleged disabled person. At this point in the proceeding, the disabled person is referred to as "alleged" because the court has not yet determined that he or she is, in fact, disabled.
- The petitioner's relationship to the alleged disabled person and interest in the person or property.
- The name and address of the person with whom the alleged disabled person resides.

- The names and addresses of all interested persons known to the petitioner and the nature of their interest. The set of interested persons includes primarily the relatives of the alleged disabled person and possibly close friends.
- A brief description of the alleged disability and the reason for seeking the guardianship.
- The specific relief sought. This provides an opportunity for the petitioner to tell the court what should be done for the person based upon the petitioner's knowledge of the person's situation. Usually the petitioner suggests a particular individual as the potential guardian. This may be the petitioner him- or herself, another relative, a close friend, or the department of social services if no one else is available. If the social services department becomes the guardian, a caseworker is assigned to the person.

Q.7:43 What additional documentation is included with the petition?

The petition must contain certificates from two physicians attesting to the disability. These certificates must be issued within a reasonable time before the petition is filed; the petitioner cannot use certificates from years ago. The period of preceding time considered reasonable may be as few as 10 days or as many as 45 days, depending upon the state law.

Each certificate must contain the qualifications of the physician, the date of the last examination of the patient, and the opinion regarding whether the patient has sufficient mental capacity to consent to the appointment of a guardian. The physician must also give an opinion about the probable duration of the disability so that the court may appoint a guardian for an appropriate term. Practically speaking, most appointments are permanent, although subject to review at any time if the condition of the disabled person improves.

Q.7:44 What due process procedures are in place for the appointment of a guardian?

Because the appointment of a guardian deprives the alleged disabled person of essential powers of decisionmaking, this person must be given ample opportunity to address the charge of disability. Several key steps must be taken:

- Service of process. The alleged disabled person must be served with a copy of the petition. The court will send the information to this person's current address.
- Order to show cause. This is an order issued by the court that directs the interested persons named in the petition to show cause (demonstrate) why a guardian should be appointed. This is the opportunity for these persons to voice their views about the guardianship itself or about the individuals who might be named as guardian.
- Appointment of an attorney. The court will appoint an attorney to represent the interests of the alleged disabled person if the person does not have his or her own attorney.
- Hearing. The court will hold a hearing to which all parties and interested persons are encouraged to come. Usually the alleged disabled person does not attend the hearing.
- Order appointing guardian. The judge will issue an order appointing the guardian. The judge will also specify duties of the guardian based upon the nature of the disability.

Q.7:45 Is a guardianship permanent?

The appointment of a guardian lasts for as long as the judge specifies in the decree. In most cases, the appointment is permanent, but it may be for a specific period of time if the disability is related to surgery or an illness with a predictable outcome. At any time,

however, that the disabled person or any interested person believes that the condition has improved to such a point that the disabled person is able to handle his or her own affairs, the court may be petitioned to terminate the guardianship of the person on the ground that the disability has ceased.

Q.7:46 May an HHA be involved as a petitioner or as a guardian?

Legally, yes. Any individual may petition the court for appointment of a guardian. If, however, a nurse or aide or other HHA staff member observes the need for such a procedure, it would be best if he or she reports it to the HHA administration. The administrator or social worker could then contact the social services department, which would file the petition on the patient's behalf.

In addition, an HHA staff member could, in theory, be appointed guardian, depending upon who else is available to assume those duties. It would be preferable to have the social services agency appoint a guardian if no family member or friend was available. It can happen, however, that an HHA nurse or aide and a patient develop a special relationship and the staff member wants to care for the patient.

The problem is that a nurse (or aide) may have information about a patient's finances or personal situation that could lead to a conflict of interest. For example, the patient may have confided financial information, and the nurse may be thinking he or she can get access to the patient's money. In fact, he or she cannot, because the nurse must account to the court each year for the expenditures on behalf of the patient. Some court systems are vigilant about this, others are open to abuse. But if an HHA staff member wants to be the guardian for a patient, he or she should no longer treat that patient. Other clinical personnel should oversee the care of the patient so that an objective view is always maintained.

Q.7:47 What specific role might HHA personnel play in a guardianship procedure?

HHA personnel may be involved in a procedure for obtaining a guardian of the person. [See Martha Dale Nathanson and Richard B.

Stofberg, "Guardianship and the Primary Care Physician," *Physician Practice Digest*, Spring 1994.] The role of such personnel, including nurses, therapists, and possibly aides, would be as witnesses to confirm that the person is in fact unable to manage his or her affairs effectively. A physician must attest, as a legal matter, that the patient is in need of a guardian. This physician must have examined the patient within a short time prior to executing the certificate. The certificate is legally sufficient evidence of the patient's need for a guardian, but in most cases the court will require further evidence, as the appointment of a guardian takes away significant decision-making rights from the patient.

The home health nurse or therapist, or even an aide if the aide has communicated with the patient frequently enough, could provide the court important information regarding the patient's situation. For example, the home health personnel may know more than the physician about the family situation and why there is allegedly no family member available to care for the patient. If the guardianship is contested by a family member or other individual, the home health personnel can shed light on the circumstances.

Q.7:48 Will HHA personnel have to go to court?

Usually the guardianship can be obtained without court appearances by any of the medical personnel. They can complete affidavits explaining their observations regarding the patient's condition and why the patient needs a guardian of the person.

If the court needs more information or wishes to ask the provider directly about the patient, the court may request the nurse or therapist or aide to appear personally at the hearing. If the staff member is not available, he or she may be asked to stand by for a telephone call from the judge during the hearing.

Regardless of whether the testimony is given in court or on the telephone, the judge will ask a few questions about the patient's history and condition and whether in the staff member's opinion the patient needs a guardian or can take care of him- or herself. The staff member should be prepared to have his or her opinion "attacked" by the attorney for the patient, as it is that attorney's job to ensure that the patient's rights are protected and removed only if absolutely necessary.

Ultimately, HHA personnel can contribute to the well-being of the patient and help ensure that his or her rights are being protected as well. In such a process, there is no "winner" or "loser," for the protection of the patient is the goal of all parties.

Q.7:49 Who may or may not be appointed a guardian of the person?

Most states provide a hierarchy of individuals who may be appointed guardian, according to their availability. The court will also examine their propriety for the task. The individuals eligible to be appointed guardian of the person are listed below in order of priority:

1. a person nominated by the disabled person if he or she had the mental capacity to make an intelligent choice at the time of the designation;
2. the disabled person's spouse;
3. the disabled person's parents;
4. a person nominated by the will of a deceased person who, during his or her life, had a relationship with the disabled person;
5. the disabled person's children;
6. adults who would be the disabled person's heirs if he or she were dead;
7. a person nominated by another person caring for the disabled person (an HHA staff member could possibly be requested by a family member or neighbor to serve as guardian); and
8. any other person considered appropriate by the court (the patient's relatives or close friends would fall into this category; the court would have notice of their availability because they would be listed on the petition as "interested persons").

PATIENT ABANDONMENT

Q.7:50 What is the general duty regarding acceptance of a patient and continuation of medical treatment?

Generally, when an individual engages a health care practitioner for purposes of treatment, presumably the intent is for the health care practitioner to treat the patient throughout the illness. Once initiated, the relationship continues until both parties agree to end it, until the patient discharges the practitioner, or until the services are no longer needed, and until that time the practitioner is under a duty to continue to provide necessary medical care to the patient. [Am. Jur. 2d Physicians and Surgeons, §234.]

In regards to an HHA providing treatment to a patient, the duty flows to the HHA, not to the individual practitioner. Thus, the HHA has no duty to provide the same nurse or physical therapist to the patient during the course of treatment as long as the treatment is undertaken consistently with the plan of care. Of course, it may be in the best interests of the HHA to send the same practitioner to the patient as consistently as possible to ensure continuity of care from a clinical perspective as well as to develop a trusting relationship between the parties to mitigate the difficulty of problems that may arise.

If the patient dismisses a particular nurse or home health aide, the HHA still has a duty to provide care, unless the patient also specifically discharges the agency itself. Supervisory personnel should always inquire as to the intent of the patient regarding the dismissal, and continue providing care until affirmatively told not to. To do otherwise may open the agency up to a charge of abandonment.

Q.7:51 What is the general definition of abandonment?

Case law generally defines abandonment as a unilateral severance of the professional relationship between doctor and patient without reasonable notice at a time when there is still the necessity of continuing medical attention. [*Lee v. Dewbre*, 362 SW 2d 900 (Tex.

Civ. App. 7th Dist. 1962).] Further, the physician is under a duty to give his or her patient all necessary and continued attention as long as the case requires it and should not leave the patient in a critical state without giving reasonable notice or making suitable arrangements for the attendance of another physician. [*Katsetos v. Nolan,* 368 A.2d 172 (Conn. 1976).]

Although the cases concern to the physician-patient relationship, the principles are applicable to all providers of medical care. In addition, the care rendered by an HHA is provided pursuant to a physician's plan of care, and thus even if in a particular case the HHA was not found liable for abandonment and the physician was, the physician would likely seek indemnification from the HHA, as it was the entity providing the services.

Q.7:52 What actions would open an HHA up to a charge of abandonment?

Many types of actions could inspire a charge of abandonment. Each action must be viewed in the context of the overall relationship between the HHA and the patient, but any of the following actions should be carefully scrutinized:

- The practitioner expressly declares that he or she withdraws from the case either without naming a successor to treat the patient or naming a successor who is not competent to treat that particular patient.
- The practitioner leaves the patient during or immediately after a procedure while his or her presence is still medically advisable.
- The practitioner fails to attend to the patient even though he or she communicated to the patient, the patient's family, or the HHA that he or she would continue to treat the patient. There need not even be an express promise to continue treatment if a promise was implied from prior continuous treatment and others would have no indication that treatment would not continue.

- The practitioner fails to give proper instructions to the patient or patient's family before leaving the home.
- The practitioner refuses to continue to treat the patient because the patient can no longer pay for services.

Even though these and similar actions may lead to a charge of abandonment, the patient may ultimately prevail only if it can be shown that the abandonment was indeed the proximate cause of an injury to the patient. Thus, if an HHA abandons a patient but the patient ultimately needed no further home health services, no injury would have occurred and no claim for abandonment will likely prevail.

Q.7:53 How can an HHA avoid the problem of patient abandonment?

First, while there is no surefire way to predict problem cases or problem patients, the HHA should carefully screen requests for home health services and not accept cases it may not be able to handle. Once treatment is undertaken, the HHA is obliged to continue providing services unless a substitute provider can be found, and, in all practicality, if one HHA cannot handle the case, chances are the case is not appropriate for any number of other agencies in the area.

All personnel should be trained to handle requests from patients responsibly. For example, if a patient vehemently tells the occupational therapist to "get out and never come back," the OT should cheerfully tell the patient that he will arrange for another OT to come next time. The OT should immediately inform the HHA that the patient has requested another OT, and the HHA should immediately assign another OT to visit the patient.

In such a situation, the HHA, through the OT or other personnel, should give or send the patient a letter explaining that the HHA is responding to his request to have another OT on the case. A copy of the letter signed by both parties should be placed in the patient's clinical record, but if that is not possible, a copy signed by the agency or at least a note should be placed in the chart reflecting the assignment of a new practitioner. A sample letter follows:

Date:

Dear:

You have requested a new occupational therapist to continue your treatment. We are happy to continue to provide you home health services and would like to introduce your new occupational therapist _____. We hope you will continue to be satisfied with our service. Please let us know if we can help you further.

[Patient Signature]   [HHA Signature]

* * * *

If the HHA wishes to terminate the relationship or the patient wishes to terminate the relationship with the agency as a whole, the HHA should inform the patient (or guardian or other caregivers) both verbally and in writing if possible, but in all cases in writing. The HHA must continue to provide care for a reasonable period of time and must offer the patient the opportunity to find a new HHA. If the patient requests, the HHA may refer the patient to another HHA capable of providing the required services to the patient. A copy of the letter of termination signed by both parties should be placed in the patient's chart. If that is not possible, the HHA should note in the chart that the patient was informed appropriately and attach a copy of the letter. A sample letter follows:

Date:

Dear:

[As you have requested,] Home Health Agency, Inc., will no longer be able to provide home health services to _____ _____. If you require home health services within the next

___ days, Home Health Agency, Inc., will provide them, but in no event for more than ___ days.

To assist you in continuing to receive medical care for _____, we will make your clinical records available to a new agency as soon as you authorize us to send them to that agency. If you do not have a particular agency in mind, we will be happy to give you a list of [Medicare-certified] agencies that you may contact for services.

[Patient signature]   [HHA signature]

[Adapted from Am.Jur. Legal Forms 2d Physicians and Surgeons §202:64, Physician's Letter of Withdrawal from Case—American Medical Association form.]

Send all required notices by certified mail, return receipt requested.

Q.7:54 Should an HHA sever its relationship with a patient if the patient wants the HHA to provide certain equipment or services that the HHA deems not appropriate for that patient?

The HHA should of course advise the patient that the equipment or services are not appropriate in the treatment of the particular condition. A staff member should carefully explain why the equipment or services are not indicated, state what the possible consequences are if they are provided as the patient requests, and suggest alternatives to the patient and explain why those alternatives are appropriate. The administrator should speak with the patient and explain again why the agency believes the patient should not receive the requested equipment or services.

If the patient still insists upon receiving the particular equipment or services and the HHA can provide them without risking negligence, the HHA can ask the patient to enter into an agreement that acknowledges the HHA has advised against the particular equipment or services and yet is willing to provide them at the patient's insistence. This type of agreement is known as a "covenant not to sue."

The document should state explicitly that discussions have occurred regarding the provision of equipment or services and the patient understands the consequences of obtaining them. By signing the document, the patient agrees not to sue the HHA in any action regarding the equipment or particular services. A sample covenant not to sue follows:

COVENANT NOT TO SUE

This Agreement is made this ___ day of _____, 19____, by and between _____, of _____, ("Customer") and The Caring Home Health Agency, and any of its affiliated, related or subsidiary entities ("Company").

Customer desires to obtain certain equipment or services from Company, and Company has advised Customer that the equipment or services are not ideal under the circumstances. Company has offered Customer a suitable alternative, but Customer still desires to utilize equipment or services against advice of Company;

Now, therefore, Customer and Company hereby agree as follows:

That Customer covenants not to sue and to forever refrain from instituting, procuring, or in any way aiding, any suit, cause of action, or claim against the Company, which Customer now believes, may in the future believe, or has in the past believed, resulted directly or indirectly from use of the specific equipment or services

_____
_____.

Further, Customer hereby agrees to hold harmless and indemnify Company against any loss or liability, claims, costs, charges, and expenses incident to any claim or claims arising out of the use of the product by the Customer, on account of any action brought by the Customer in violation of this agreement at any time before or after this agreement is signed.

This instrument is not intended to accomplish a release of a cause of action arising on account of any damages to the Customer, but is intended only as a covenant not to sue, expressly reserving to the

Customer all rights to proceed against any persons or entities other than the Company for any claim or demand arising out of the use of the product listed above.

IN WITNESS WHEREOF, the Customer has signed this Covenant Not To Sue on this _____ day of _____, 19___ , at _____.

[WITNESS]:   [Customer Signature]

                                             [Company Signature]

Q.7:55 What is the difference between a covenant not to sue and a general release?

A general release serves to release *all* possible claims against any parties, not just against one particular party, for particular services.

8

Recordkeeping

An essential part of any business is the documentation that reflects the manner in which the business has provided its product to consumers. A home health agency must keep records for financial reasons as well as for quality assurance purposes. In some instances, clinical records will need to be changed to reflect changes in a patient's status, and the agency must ensure that changes are made properly. In addition, employment laws require certain records to be kept, and the agency must set up systems to track employee issues. An agency's records can serve it well in helping it manage its patients, its finances, and its employees, and spending the time and money to ensure that the recordkeeping systems are set up properly is well worth the investment.

Q.8:1 What types of records are HHAs required to keep?

The two primary types of records that HHAs must keep are clinical records and employment-related records.

CLINICAL RECORDS

Q.8:2 What are clinical records?

Clinical records, also known as medical records, can be defined any number of ways. For example, one state statute defines a "medical record" as

> any oral, written, or other transmission of information that
> is
> - written in the record of a patient or recipient;
> - identifies or can readily be associated with the identity of a
>   patient or recipient;
> - and relates to the health care of the patient or recipient. [Md.
>   Code Ann. Health General Article §4-301.]

Although this definition clearly covers actual clinical records maintained in a facility, it also covers less structured formats, such as minutes from case conferences or notes recorded by clinicians outside the official record and inserted into the record.

Another state statute takes a different approach:

> "Medical record" means any document or combination of
> documents, except births, deaths, and the fact of admission
> to or discharge from a hospital, that pertains to the medical
> history, diagnosis, prognosis, or medical condition of a
> patient and that is generated and maintained in the process
> of medical treatment. [Ohio Revised Statutes §149.42.]

The Medicare program describes the contents of an HHA clinical record. It must contain appropriate identifying information, including the name of the physician; the patient's drug, dietary treatment, and activity orders; signed and dated clinical and progress notes; and copies of summary reports sent to the attending physician.

The Joint Commission on the Accreditation of Healthcare Organizations (Joint Commission) applies certain standards for the creation and maintenance of medical records. The basic standard is that the medical record must be confidential, secure, current, authenticated, legible, and complete. The quality of the medical record, according to the Joint Commission, depends upon the timeliness, meaningfulness, authentication, and legibility of the informational content. Therefore, all entries must be dated and authenticated. The medical record must contain sufficient information to identify the patient, support the diagnosis, justify the treatment, and document the course and results accurately.

Q.8:3 How long must an HHA retain its records?

For purposes of Medicare reimbursement, clinical records must be maintained for five years after the month the cost report to which the records apply is filed with the intermediary, unless state law specifies a longer period of time. The HHA must arrange for retention of the records even if the HHA discontinues its operations. If the patient enters a health care facility, the HHA must send a copy of the home health clinical record with the patient. Although the regulation does not explicitly state this, presumably the HHA could send it directly to the facility.

Q.8:4 Are clinical records reviewed?

Appropriate health professionals must review a sample of both active and closed clinical records at least quarterly to determine whether established policies are being followed in furnishing services directly or under arrangement. Every 62 days, if the patient is still receiving home health services, the clinical record must be reviewed to assess adequacy of the plan of care and appropriateness of continuation of care. [42 C.F.R. §484.52.]

Q.8:5 Who makes entries into the records?

The HHA should be very specific about which employees are allowed to make entries into the medical record. Certainly the physician and registered nurse should be authorized to record observations, diagnoses, and treatment notes. In addition, the various types of therapists, including speech, physical, and occupational therapists, should be able to enter notes in the clinical record.

The HHA should review, however, whether licensed practical nurses and home health aides should be allowed to enter notes. On the one hand, their contact with patients may be more regular than that of the other parties, and thus their observations and recommendations can make a substantial contribution to appropriate care. On the other hand, it might be too risky to have a large number of individuals allowed access to the records. If it is decided to deny nurses and aides access, they should be encouraged to express their insights and concerns in a different manner. For example, their views can be heard at regular patient care conferences, and the HHA should create an atmosphere in which they feel free to bring up issues as they arise.

Q.8:6 May a patient or other individuals besides medical personnel see the patient's medical record?

Yes, but the HHA should have procedures controlling disclosure that accurately reflect any state law on the subject. For example, Maryland defines disclosure as "the transmission or communication of information in a medical record, including an acknowledgement that a medical record on a particular patient or recipient exists." [Md. Code Ann. Health General Article §§4-301 *et seq.*] In order for any individual, including the patient or any "person in interest" authorized by law, to receive information, that person must request in writing to see or to copy the record.

A "person in interest" is a statutory term whose definition covers the following:

- an adult on whom a medical record is kept;
- a person authorized to consent to health care for an adult;
- a duly appointed representative of a deceased individual;
- a minor or a minor's parent, guardian, or other representative; and
- an attorney appointed by any of the above individuals.

Generally, a provider must keep the fact of the existence of a medical record as well as its contents confidential. This requirement protects the patient against inquiries by unauthorized persons. If the HHA receives an inquiry regarding a patient's record, the HHA should not indicate that there is a medical record until the HHA is certain that the request is from an authorized individual.

Q.8:7 In what other situations may an HHA disclose records?

An HHA may disclose records without authorization from a person in interest for the purpose of obtaining payment, to legal counsel for the purpose of handling a claim against the HHA, to health care employees who need the information to provide services to the patient, and for research regarding more efficient means of health care delivery, or accreditation purposes. [See Md. Code Ann. Health General Article §§4-305, 4-306.]

To implement this provision, an HHA should obtain consent for release of the patient's clinical record for two particular purposes at the time the patient initiates services. First, the consent should authorize the HHA to release information to third-party payers, including Medicare, about services rendered to the patient for the purpose of obtaining payment from that third-party payer for those services.

In addition, the HHA's consent form should authorize the agency to release information to governmental and private agencies performing quality assurance activities. For example, the Joint Commission will want to review patient records in performing its accreditation survey. State departments of health may also want to see such records during inspections for certification. The most practical way to effect the release of information is to ask the patient to sign a consent narrowly drawn for these two purposes upon the initiation of services rather than having to follow up at the time disclosure actually becomes necessary.

Q.8:8 If an HHA needs to alter a clinical record, how should the change be made?

In general, patients' medical records should be maintained as originally created and should not be modified. There are, however, situations in which modifying a record may be necessary. For example, if the physician changes the patient's diagnosis or adds new symptoms related to a previous diagnosis, a switch to a new third-party payer may need to be noted. If it is necessary to change the record, it should be done in specific ways. [See Martha Dale Nathanson, "A Safe Method for Alteration of Medical Records," *Physician Practice Digest*, Spring 1992.]

First of all, the HHA should limit the number and types of personnel who are permitted to change a record. Access to the records for this purpose should be limited to clinical personnel. The HHA might want to designate physicians and certain nurses, perhaps those involved in quality assurance and risk management activities, as they would be more attuned to the need to make changes carefully.

All personnel should observe the following procedures when making any changes to a clinical record:

- When adding to a record, note any later observations chronologically in the record referring to the original entry. Also note at the original entry that additional observations are recorded later.

- Never completely mark out previously recorded notations. Instead, draw a single line through an incorrect entry, enter the correct information, initial the correction, and record the time and date of entry. These changes might read as follows:

poorly JD

January 20. Patient walking ~~steadily~~ after surgery due to fracture of the right femur.

(See note ahead, Jan. 24)

January 24. Fracture was to the left femur, not the right. John Doe, M.D., 12:30 p.m.

(see prior note, Jan. 20).

- It might also be helpful to circle the new entry so that it is clear that it has been inserted into the record.

Q.8:9 What if the patient wishes to have a change made to the medical record?

If a person in interest, including but not limited to the patient, wishes to make a change to the record, the HHA must allow that change or notify the person in writing why the change cannot be made. The HHA should allow the person to insert into the record a reason why he or she disagrees with the record. No deletions may be made, only changes or additions. If the HHA discloses any portion of the record after an addition, correction, or notice of disagreement has been made, the HHA must include a copy of such change with the record. [Md. Code Ann. Health General Article §4-304.]

Q.8:10 What are the potential consequences of improperly altering a medical record?

A clinician could be subject to prosecution under federal and state laws governing medical records. In addition, the clinician's license could be revoked for failure to keep adequate medical records. One Florida court censured a physician for making later entries into a record without properly noting that they were not part of the original record, charging that the physician had made "deceptive, untrue and fraudulent representations in the practice of medicine." [See *Jimenez v. Dept. of Professional Regulation*, 556 So.2d 1219 (Fla. App. 4th Dist. 1990).]

Insurers may also attempt to withdraw liability coverage if they learn that medical records have been altered improperly, based upon the argument that they cannot present a proper defense if the records appear to have been falsified. An HHA's Joint Commission accreditation might also be threatened if it does not maintain records according to the Joint Commission's stated standards. Finally, should an HHA or any of its employees end up on the wrong end of a lawsuit, an incident of altering a medical record without proper notification in the record could turn the case against them.

EMPLOYMENT RECORDS

Q.8:11 What types of employment records must an HHA keep?

Although an employer is not required to maintain a separate personnel file, many federal employment laws require an employer to develop and maintain certain records in order for the appropriate government agencies to be able to enforce the laws. A summary of these requirements follows:

- The Fair Labor Standards Act requires employers to maintain wage records for at least three years. The records must contain basic personal information, such as name, address, date of birth, gender, and occupation, and all payroll-related information. This information must also be kept for purposes of the Equal Pay Act, as must any additional information needed to substantiate any higher wages paid to one gender.
- Title VII of the Civil Rights Act does not require any specific records, but employment-related records that the employer keeps as a matter of course must be maintained for at least six months from their creation. Employers with at least a hundred employees must complete and file the Standard Form 100 (Employer Information Report—EEO-1) annually.
- The Age Discrimination in Employment Act requires all employment-related records to be kept for three years, including recruitment records, promotion and demotion records, tests and scores, and physical examination results.
- The Occupational Safety and Health Act requires employers to record workplace accidents and to maintain medical records and records of exposure to toxic substances during the term of the employment and for 30 years after employment is terminated. OSHA also requires employers to maintain records indicating compliance with bloodborne pathogen standards.
- The Immigration Reform and Control Act requires each employee to complete a I-9 form at the time of recruitment. It also requires the employer to keep the I-9 for three years in the case

of individuals not hired and for three years after hire or one year after termination, whichever is later, in the case of individuals hired.

- The Employee Polygraph Protection Act requires records of polygraph tests to be retained for three years after the test.

Q.8:12 If an HHA maintains personnel files for employees, must the employees have access to their files?

Some states have laws requiring employers to allow an employee to review his or her own personnel file, but regardless of whether or not employers are required to disclose such files, an HHA should have a policy addressing this issue. Basically, access should be limited to documents that the employee has completed or signed and that include no information about any other employees or other agency business. This policy protects the privacy of other employees and protects the agency against charges of invasion of privacy.

Documents that fall into the category described above include, but are not limited to, the following:

- employment application;
- employment offer and acceptance letters;
- performance appraisals and related documents;
- disciplinary documentation;
- employment contracts and related agreements addressing non-disclosure of confidential information and noncompetition; and
- separation or discharge documentation.

Index

Note: Numbers indicate chapter and question numbers not page numbers (e.g., 1:3
  indicates Chapter 1, question 3).

About the Author _____

Martha Dale Nathanson, EdS, JD, is the corporate Director of Risk Management and Regulatory Affairs for the Kirson Medical Equipment Company, headquartered in Baltimore, Maryland. Her work involves a variety of legal and operational matters, including traditional and managed care contracting, ensuring regulatory compliance, employment-related matters, Medicare and other third-party reimbursement, legislative and regulatory activity at the state and national levels, and risk management activities, including monitoring clinical compliance, insurance management, and training. Prior to her current position, Ms. Nathanson held a position as an associate at Ober, Kaler, Grimes and Shriver (a law firm with a specialty in health care), served with the Health Care Financing Administration, and worked in employment management at an urban medical center. She holds the Juris Doctor degree and the Specialist in Education from Indiana University at Bloomington.

Ms. Nathanson is currently Chair of the Licensure Committee of the National Association of Medical Equipment Services and Chair of the Legislative Committee of the Medical Equipment Dealers of Maryland. She is an active member of the Forum on Home Care Issues, a coalition addressing the integration of the various elements of the home care field. She is a regular contributor on legal matters to the *Physician Practice Digest*, a publication for members of the Maryland, District of Columbia, and Virginia medical societies.